Health Guide

Master Beinsa Douno

ISBN-13: 978-1489537447
ISBN-10: 1489537449

CONTENTS

Way Of Life in Accordance with the Laws of Animate Nature (Prevention)

MASTER BEINSA DOUNO

HUMAN BODY

Structure

Everything, created by God, also exists in miniature in man.

Each man is a string of God's instrument and Rational creatures play on it by their bows.

Man's body is a result of God's energy. It has created the present human organism.

Man has 12 bodies, but only four function for the present: the physical one; the one of the heart (feelings); the third one is the one of the mind, and the fourth one – of the rational, causal world.

The other eight bodies are in an embryonic state. They will manifest themselves in future. When you enter the Spiritual world, four more will manifest themselves, and when you enter in the Divine world, the other four will develop.

Man's soul has its special body, with which it can ascend. This body is so plastic and so well made that it can become both - small or big. Exactly that body builds also the physical one and all the rest man's bodies.

Body is as important as the mind and heart. It is an environment, and soil, from which we obtain the powers of life.

The body is a Divine garment, which renovates itself constantly. Body changes every seven years. Thanks to this constant exchange, man feels healthy and bright.

The spiritual body is being built at the moment. It is not completed. The forehead, the nose, the mouth, the hairs, the cranium, the mind, the hands are not completed. The astral arm is being developed now. The astral world is getting dense. It is preparing for a higher and more purified life life. At the moment it is in something like water state.

Man is cone-like in form: up, at the shoulders, he is wider, and down – he is narrower. This shows descending of man to the physical, i.e. material world.

Man's head is a result of the cultures, through which man has passed as a human being. His body is a result of animal cultures, a result of animal activity. Matter is a result of plant's activity. When he was in the phase of a plant, man created the materials for building of his body. When he was in the phase of an animal, he created his body and when he came to the phase of a human being, he created his head and face. God drew a breath in man and he became a living creature.

The matter, of which man is created, is different from the matter of all other animals and creatures.

The forms, of which one animal is created, are of special powers; of special matter. That matter cannot be so easily transformed. Each man is created of special type of matter. There is more gold in the blood of some people, and in others – more silver, and in third people – iron, in fourth people – copper, etc. The gold in the blood is no more than one ten-millionth part of milligram, but it influences man's character. If scientists want to find that gold through the scales, which they have, they will never find it, but in the blood of some people it exists and its influence is powerful. There is a type of matter and if we had from it in our bodies, we would have done wonders. The original matter, of which the world is created, was a thousand times more diluted than hydrogen. The original powers, which have functioned in that matter, were so strong that if it were possible to be obtained only one gram of it at present, all industrial enterprises, which exist all over the world, would have worked day and night for three thousand years.

According to the occult science, the matter, of which man is created, is not taken only from the the Earth. That matter, of which man is created, initially the space man, is taken from the whole Universe, from all Suns and planets per one small part and today's body is put together.

On the grounds of what part from the planet we have taken, that matter is connected to us and it influences us. The type of influence on us in physical and psychic respect depends on what and how much matter we have taken from the planets.

The better, more rational and stronger man is, the stronger and finer his organs are made. His matter is finer and of better quality. Such a man is called healthy and organized. The structure of man's external and internal organs corresponds to the powers of his organism in the way, in which clothes correspond to man's internal qualities and culture.

Organs of human organism are created by popular virtues. Hence each disease of any of the organs influences that virtue, which creates the relevant organ.

Do you know how many creatures suffer and give their lives, in order human body to be maintained?! That is why you do not have the right to think that what you have is yours. All that you have is not yours. All that you have is not yours, but God's. You shall say: "God, thank You for putting me inside that body of Yours. "

Each organ has a double service: external and internal, i.e. material and spiritual.

Truth, in its simplest form, is necessary for the restoration of the balance in the organism: it keeps the digestive system in good form. Justice shall lie in the base of the heart and make man healthy. Justice keeps the heart and the lungs in good working order. There is melancholy, where justice is missing.

Man is normally developed if there is a regular proportion between the height and width, between the arms and legs, between the head, trunk and limbs. By all means there must be a certain proportion between the figures, which define the separate parts of the human body. If one of these figures changes, the rest change simultaneously.

If man knows how to think, he can make, he can build one perfect body and one beautiful perfect face.

The feet of the legs, in a normally developed man or woman, shall be 1/6 part of the height; the face shall be 1/10 part of the height; the chest-1/4; the length of the arm till the wrist - 1/10.

Forehead is a measure, with which God measures. Nose is a measure, with which angles measure. Chin is a measure, with which man measures.

Man's eyebrows shall be as long as the nose. Mouth shall be as big as the eyebrows. These are measures, taken from Nature.

Generally, the upper part of man, and particularly the chests, shall be wide, and the waist and abdomen shall be delicate, thin.

The wider man's brain is, the greater his endurance in the physical world is. The width of the brain corresponds to the width of female thighs. The length of the brain corresponds to male shoulders. People with wide shoulders are male no matter if they are in female or male form. A woman with broad shoulders is more male than female. A man with broad thighs is more female than male.

Present man's conscious functions in the physical body, in the astral body, in the mental and causal bodies. There are other bodies in man, but they are stagnant. There some organs in the physical body, which correspond to ones in the other bodies. For example, the brain corresponds to the mental body. The sympathetic nervous system or the stomach brain corresponds to the spiritual body. The liver, spleen and stomach correspond to the lower fields of the astral body. If the liver is in bad condition, the feelings will not function properly; you will be in dark moods, indisposed. Liver helps digestion and if the poisons, which have appeared, do not go to the stomach, the will go into the blood and will cause misbalance in the astral body. Then the powers of the astral body will not go properly into the physical body. If the liver is in bad shape, brain fades. After that neurasthenia comes, because this organ influences indirectly the sympathetic nervous system. If any of the functions of an organ worsens, this influences the others, too. If you do not control your feelings, they will upset the liver, and the liver will misbalance your whole organism.

Each element has a definite place in the human body: for example the place of oxygen is in man's blood; of the nitrogen – in the brain, in the nervous system; of the hydrogen – in the stomach; of the carbon – in the bones.

All organs in man are created in accordance with his character, in accordance with his soul. Man's body is the same as his soul. Man's eyes are the same as his mind. Man's mouth is the same as his heart. Man's nose is the same as his intelligence. Man's legs are the same as his virtues. Man's justice is the same as his arms.

The function of the stomach system in the physical world is to digest food, and in the spiritual world – to decompose man's lusts and lower desires through digestion; to cut them up into small pieces and send them upwards to the hearth. In the physical world, the heart and lungs purify the blood, and in the spiritual – they are the bellows and the hearth, through which man's desires have to pass, in order the clean to be separated from the unclean. The brain system addresses its orders to the various organs for the service, which they have to perform. In the spiritual world, the brain defines the service and the place of all thoughts in man. Do not mix the clean thoughts with the unclean ones. Thinking is connected to the desires, and desires – to the actions, and the actions – to the consequences.

Brain, as well as the heart and lungs have a dual function: physiological and psychic. The heart purifies not only the blood, but also the feelings. Lungs purify not only the air, but they are an altar, where man's thoughts, feelings and desires are being purified. The sacred fire, which purifies and strengthens things, burns on this alter.

Each organ, each system in man has a relation to his life. For example, the stomach has a relation to man's physical world. When he arranges his material matters, his stomach will work well. When he messes them up, his stomach upsets. It is noticed that man can be physically healthy without being strong. Hence strength comes from somewhere else. From where does man's strength come? From lungs. Strong man is the one, who breaths in a right way. On the other hand, the stomach delivers the needed materials for building of the human body, i.e. the one of the physical man. When a house is being built, before starting its building, small sheds are built, in which woods, lime, etc. are stored. The stomach may be compared namely to those sheds. The building materials are being stored in it, which are distributed later to the entire organism.

Man connects to cherubim through lungs. That is why, when you breathe, think about that spirits and their wisdom. Hence wisdom is adopted through breathing. Man connects to another hierarchy, called "thrones", i.e. Divine mind, through his heart. Heart's beat shows that we are connected to that hierarchy. Man is connected to other hierarchies of creatures of nobleness through the stomach. That is why, when man is fed, he becomes more disposed, better, nobler and ready for sacrifices. From the stomach, it is reached the liver, through which man connects to another hierarchy, called "powers" or Divine power. Through the gall man is connected to the creatures of good. When the gall is in good condition, goodness and love increase. If hatred increases, love decreases. That is a law, which regulates the relations between the powers. No one can avoid that law. Spleen, through which man connects to another hierarchy - "principalities", called Divine justice and victory in the world, comes after the liver. Another hierarchy are the archangels – creatures of God's glory. They rule peoples. They have a relation to the kidneys. Finally we reach to the hierarchy of the angels, which are the basis of life.

Today thinking manifests itself through brain, feelings – through the sympathetic nervous system, in the so called solar plexus, which is incorrectly called heart. Will is manifested through arms and legs.

Three factors take part in man's nourishment. The first factor is the stomach. It delivers the material food for the entire organism. The second factor is the lungs, which intake the air through the mouth and purifies, i.e. oxygenises the blood through it. The third factor is the brain, which sends the energies all over the body.

Digestion influences the circulation; the circulation – the respiratory system; the respiratory system – the nervous system, and the nervous system – the brain – headquarters of thinking. The brain and nervous system are not at the place, where thoughts are created. They just perceive and process thoughts. There is one high world, where thoughts are created and send to our world through the brain and nervous system, which are conductors of those thoughts.

The principle of the mind is determined by the brain nervous system, in which the brain, nerves and human senses play main roles. The principle of the heart or the power of sensitivity is connected to his respiratory, circulatory and digestive systems. Man's will, which is determined by his most supreme ability – the mind, is a power, which manifests itself through the motor system. Man is sensible only when he knows how to use the various parts of his body.

The multiple world is man's head. The spiritual world is his lungs, his heart, which beats and moves blood, and the human stomach is the physical, the material world. Hence man shall know that he lives in the three worlds simultaneously.

Man distinguishes from all animals by his head. It represents the first world. His second world begins from the neck, involves the chest with the heart, the lungs and a part of the stomach. The third world begins from the stomach downwards and involves the intestines, the liver and kidneys.

The physical world is man's stomach, which is composed of three zones: hell - large intestines, purgatory – small intestines, and paradise – the stomach itself.

The spiritual world is the lungs, composed of two wings: a right one, through which good passes, and a left one, through which evil passes. The right wing of the lungs is paradise, and the left one - hell.

Man's head, in which the brain is, is the Divine world. The front part of the head – the forehead and the upper part, are the good, the paradise in man. The back part of the head is the hell in man. Hence man lives simultaneously in the physical, spiritual and Divine worlds.

Health depends on a law, on a gland, which is in the pit of the stomach. If you connect that gland to the solar energy, if you know when this favourable energies flow away, you will have results. Each man, who can put this gland of his into contact with the solar energies, he can live on the Earth as much as he wants. And if he wants to develop his mind, he shall connect that gland to the light energies, which come from the Moon and the energies, which exist in the brain, because the energy, which is kept by the brain, is from a totally different sphere. Man's mind can be of service to him only in this world. We know the other world by our hearts. What mind knows might be true for this world, but what mind thinks about the other world is not true. What heart thinks about the internal world is true. That is why we shall study the spiritual world through the power of our hearts.

The first thing noticed in our organisms is that there is an order in them, mutuality during the common activity and harmony between all workers, who know their activities very well. Private goals are not pursued in organism. One common goal is pursued there – one common welfare, which makes man happy. The secret of the mutual success is here. There is no self-will in that organism. There are no random acts. Unity rules in it. And when one of the neighbour cells gets ill and suffers, all other cells sympathize and are in a hurry to eliminate evil in any way. Everything inside man is distributed by mathematical preciseness and as long as it exists, the powers in the organism balance each other and form that harmony, which we call health.

The prevailing character features give the form of the ear, the form of the eyes, of the eyebrows, of the hair – thin or thick, of the fingers – short or long.

The composition of the saliva changes every minute and defines the changes that happen in man's psyche. This is a science, which will be studied in future.

In one of his messages Paul says: "I service to sin by my flesh and to the law of Love - by my soul. Who will rescue me from that situation?" No one will rescue him. He will serve both his flesh and his soul.

As long as you have flesh, you will eat, sleep, and work.

As long as you have soul, you will work with it in the spiritual and in the Divine worlds.

Voluntarily or by force, man serves both his flesh and his soul.

It does not matter what is said and what is written in the sacred books. It is not possible man to get rid of his nature. The struggle between flesh and soul has always existed and will exist. Life of soul and life of flesh, no matter how opposed to each other they are, are in an equal way necessary for the human development.

Without the life of the flesh, there will be no development. Do not be afraid of flesh, but try to make it be of service to the spirit. Train your flesh in each respect.

According to the Hindus "akasha" is something, which fills the entire space and exists eternally. All forms are created of it. It is something that stands still at one place. It looks like a great aristocrat, who does not work, but always rests. The second essence is "prana", which exists eternally. This is the power, from which electricity and magnetism come out. It creates their forms. Ether, air, water, comets, all planets come out from prana and akasha. Something else, which we do not know what it is, what its essence is, stand behind prana and akasha. In order man to get benefit of prana, he shall study its laws, because various diseases like headache, tuberculosis, bad digestion, etc. come out from bad distribution of prana in human body.

If it is not well distributed in muscles, rheumatism fever occurs.

The science of prana aims at distributing that energy equally between all organs and cells, in order they not to suffer. Man cannot have healthy organism if he does not understand the laws of prana. With regard to this, breathing is nothing else, but a major method for accumulation of prana. Why shall man do things in a right way? In order he to gather prana and use it in a right way.

If mind, heart and will do not work in the way they have to, you will be deprived of the prana, which you need.

Nervous System

When we study the physiology of the nervous system, we come to the conclusion that the nervous system is an installation, through which the powers of the animate nature pass. The nervous threads are living cells – conductors of nervous energy. It passes through them in the same way as water passes through the water-conduits. If water is sandy, sand gradually settles along the pipes till one day they are completely blocked. Water installation is blocked in this way. Such blocking happens also in man's nervous system. What shall be done? You shall unblock. You shall know what types of thoughts and desires to let inside yourselves.

Man is a tree, composed of other two other trees. These two trees compose the two major systems in man: the brain one and the sympathetic nervous system. The branches of the brain system spread downwards till the limbs of the body, and the roots are up in the brain. The other tree is the stomach brain or the so called sympathetic nervous system, which consists of a raw of knots, ganglions, located mainly in the zone of the stomach. The roots of the sympathetic nervous system are planted in the ganglions, i.e. in the stomach brain, and the branches go upwards. Hence the branches of these two trees are entangled.

What is the difference between these two systems? The difference is the results from them. The brain system bears electricity and that is why if it develops more than the other one, man begins to get dry. The electricity takes out the entire moisture from the organism and that is why man is dry, without moisture. He is waterless. The sympathetic nervous system distinguishes by results opposite to the ones of the brain system. It bears man's magnetism. When it is developed in somebody, he gets fat. Excessive energy is accumulated, which afterwards transfers to fat. Hence these two systems can correct each other.

The headquarters of consciousness is in the head, and partially in the backbone. It manifests itself by the cerebrum and the spinal cord. The old capital of consciousness was somewhere else, and not in the head. There are more powers of consciousness, which are not moved to head. Where was the place of consciousness before? In the sympathetic nervous system or in the so called solar plexus. Long ago man's head was there. He thought through the solar plexus.

Man's success, in each respect, depends on the sympathetic nervous system. Joy, good-will, inspiration depend on it. This was known long ago, but it has been forgotten and shall be studied again. Today it is worked on the organization of man's heart, of man's brain. All organs are being organized now, in order to come into agreement with the sympathetic nervous system. The Divine energy comes from the sympathetic nervous system. Man's spiritual power is in the solar plexus, which I call a life-giving brain of life. The unorganized brain and the life-giving brain of life shall harmonize. This is necessary, because you belong, except to the world, in which you live, to a sublime world, too. Man's power is hidden in the sympathetic nervous system, that is why do not leave it opened for known and unknown people to come into and go out of it. Keep it closed by nine keys, but build through it nine faucets in order all who are thirsty to drink from them. The sympathetic nervous system perceives the truth and reality in a straight way and the brain just reflects them. It does not get upset, but when the flows, which come from it to the brain, are interrupted, the function of both systems is destroyed. Hatred destroys the correct activity of both systems. For rejuvenation, make exercises for about 1520 minutes for the sympathetic nervous system every day.

In the sympathetic nervous system roots of life are hidden. When conditions are established for the development of the roots, man gets fat. One, who is thin and dry, thinks more, and one, who is fat, feels more.

If we investigate the sympathetic nervous system, we will see that the roots are in the stomach, where there are glands, called stomach brain, the branches of which go into the cerebrum and from there they send their energies downwards. If the sympathetic nervous system were not managed by the cerebrum, man would have get into animal state under the law of the instinct of self-preservation.

The physical heart of man is a little to the left, and his spiritual heart is in the pit of his stomach. This place is also called solar plexus. This is the most tender zone, which one shall keep carefully.

The solar plexus is under the influence of the liver that is why one shall keep it in perfect working order. How shall it be kept in good working order? Through the solar plexus. The whole waste from the mental world and from the heart one of man goes into the liver, and from there – into the centre of the Earth, where it is purified. In this sense, the solar plexus serves as a channel for purification of unclean thoughts and feelings. One's health depends on the well-being of the liver.

The internal heart, not the one that moves the blood, but the one, in which feelings occur, is called a solar plexus. This solar plexus is an organ, which gathers the solar energy. Mind is an organ, which gathers the energy from the Moon and all other planets and stars, stores the light and makes the fine materials, the images of thinking.

In order to adopt an occult knowledge, in its sublime degree, one shall have a strong nervous system, to endure. Rough thoughts, feelings and acts influence badly the human organism. In the same way, sublime thoughts and feelings require strong nervous system.

Brain

When it is talked about the Divine world, about a higher culture, we have in mind the human brain. The Divine world is an organized world, as a result of which, changes almost do not happen in it. The same can be said about the human brain. The smallest changes happen in the human brain. It does not become weak like the body. The substance of human brains distinguishes with great stability. The biggest capital is put in the brain. On its behalf, brain has created the face. The state of the brain is recognized by the face. It is also recognized by the eyes, ears, sense of smell and taste. If we know the state of the brain we will know the state of the entire body.

The brain and the nervous system are not at the place, where thoughts are created. They only perceive and process thoughts. Hence, there is a high world, where thoughts are created and from there they are sent into our world through the brain and the nervous system, which are conductors of that thoughts.

Faith forms a hormone in you. If your faith cannot attract blood to the brain, it is weak. Hope has a special hormone, too. If your hope cannot attract blood to the brain, it is weak. If your sense cannot attract blood to your brain, it is also weakly developed. It is the same with music. Music shall attract blood to the musical centre. All centres of the human brain shall be welded by blood, in order they to be able to develop and renovate. When all centres and glands in the brain develop and renovate, then the new man is created. In the glands with internal secretion is hidden the reason for rejuvenation and even for immortality. Immortality is put into man, but he does not know how to find it. Rationality is put in man, but he does not know how to use it. All gifts are put in man, but he does not know how to develop them.

In the same way, in which a gardener waters vegetables in the garden, man shall direct his thinking toward all brain centres, push energy toward them, feed them. If he waters only some of the centres, and abandons others, he develops partially. People are unhappy, because there are partially developed.

Hunger is due to the feeling of willingness. The centre of that feeling is around the temporal zone of the brain; the more this centre is developed, the greater is the desire for food. Man shall eat, but he shall know how to eat.

Some scientists, some occultists notice that in human brain white threads begin to form. The forms of certain new organs for the future new mankind come into being. While new organs are not created in people, many things will remain unexplained to them. New people have to be created of new matter.

There are special cells in the brain, which perceive the solar light in all ranges, which are 52. We perceive only two. Other cells perceive the energies of the Earth. There are cells in the brain, which perceive science, fourth ones – arts, music; fifth ones are cells of intuition, etc. All these cells distinguish with great intelligence.

In human body the least insensible organ is brain. You can push it wherever you want, it feels nothing. But if excessive energy accumulates in it, it begins to suffer.

Once man worked with the right hemisphere and that is why the left hand has worked more. Now, as the right hemisphere has tired, work has gone to the left one and that is why man works by his right hand.

The Rational creatures, who lead the mankind, have made people work through their left hemispheres and right hands.

Some people are born with good memory, because a series of generations have worked before them and have handed it down.

Each man is born with the possibility to develop his memory. People with lower foreheads have better memories than those with higher foreheads, because the latter undertake lots of things and are frequently absent-minded.

Brain is composed of two types of matter: physical, which decomposes and spiritual (empyreal), which does not decompose. All human thoughts are imprinted on the spiritual matter of the brain. When one dies, he takes with him exactly that matter. That brain gives the image to the one that has departed.

The entire surfaces of the human brain and of the human body are perceivers of various energies, which come from everywhere, from the entire Nature.

Brain never gets ill. The reason for an eventual illness is hidden somewhere else. Brain is stable. The brain of one per ten thousand ill people may happen to be really ill and it is the back part of the brain, which will be ill, which will be due to a conflict between mind and heart.

Cells

Life comes from the Great, from the infinity, which has no a beginning and an ending. Life comes from an essence, but not from the small, but from the big. Scientists say that life has come from one small cell, and actually this cell is only a conductor of life in the way faucets are conductors of water. However, the faucet itself does not give water. Water comes from a totally another source. The cell is only a conductor of life, but an intelligent conductor. Some cells build the brain, others – the stomach, third ones – the lungs, forth ones – the nervous system, etc. They are excellent chemists. They know how to combine elements. They are smarter even than the one, in whom they are located. Man is considered to be a master of his body, and actually some of his servants know more than their master. The master should turn to God by the words: "God, I would like to know at least as much as my servants in my head know". Man shall be a little more humble and admit that he does not know much. If his life does not go well, if his blood is not clean, what does man know?

What is man? A sum of milliards of small souls or creatures, which have agreed, in the name of God's love, to enter in man and work for him and give him an appearance of a person. They have sacrificed their lives for him. They have become his servants and when he does not understand them, he says: "What is the body? It is nothing else than a machine."

There is one rational matter in the world, which penetrates into all cells all over the body, of which we even do not imagine. Round this matter, which is rational, there is a rational power, which surrounds them both. That rational matter and that rational power surround externally all cells and penetrate through all smallest particles of our organisms.

In human organism, there is one immortal cell - the original one, which everybody shall find. It is the ancestor of all cells. This original living cell distinguishes from the others by the fact that it contains horny substance in itself. The nourishing materials in it are more than in the other cells, and thanks to the horny substance, it differs with great stability. It can stand even the worst conditions.

There are specific cells in the human body, which perform the duties of the best doctors. If we get ill and leave ourselves to those cells, they can cure us. They have a laboratory, where they prepare their medications and thanks to them they perfectly heal our wounds.

Human organism is composed of approximately 60 trillion cells, which distinguish with great intelligence. All of these cells include in themselves qualities and abilities of creatures of a different culture and intelligence. For example, some of the cells of the human organism bear in themselves the culture of the plants. Some of them know well chemistry, physics. Others are excellent agronomists. They choose the conditions, at which they shall develop. They know which type of soil is good for them and which is not. There are cells, which know the laws of crystallisation. Third ones have passed through the culture of fish, birds, and mammals. Finally, there are cells, which have passed through the culture of highly advanced, rational creatures. Today these cells form the human brain.

Man distinguishes by his head. If you remove man's head, from there downwards, he looks like an animal. Thanks to his head, man has gradually separated from the other animals.

The structure of the Sun and the structure of the cells are similar. The Sun has in itself 3 zones: one of them prepares the energy, the second one – accumulates and transforms it, and the third one – sends it to the Earth. There are 3 zones in cells, too: external one, which perceives the solar energy; middle one, which accumulates it in itself, and internal one, which transforms it and turns it into a vital power. Those three zones can be also found in the human organism in a more developed form. They are most distinctive in the embryo. The external case is called ectoderm, the middle one – mesoderm, and the internal one - endoderm.

Those cells, which stop performing their duties and become harmful for the health of the other cells, are thrown away by the body in the name of the common wealth. Our health rests on that protective law of Nature.

Present people do not know that there is conscious in cells. Sometimes there is such intelligence in them, of which people do not even imagine. Your health, your abilities depend exactly on your cells. That is why, each morning, send by one good thought to all cells of yours. The Writ says: "We are a temple and God lives in us and everything in us is alive!"

God's spirit has worked on us and has given us one organism with legs, arms, a brain, a heart, etc. If we, during the present life, cannot control our organism with its powers, this brain, this heart, these nerves, arteries and all cells, what do we expect then? You wake up in the morning and think nothing about your body. Say a prayer for it. Send a thought of yours to your body. Think of all your cells, which are in your brain and stomach. Think of all living creatures, which work in it and send them, as good masters do for their servants, one thought, one blessing. Encourage them. Give them powers and they will rejoice. Speak to them. They understand everything. There is one Divine law, which rules them. Encourage them. They are Rational creatures. Be sensible and careful toward them. Speak to them as a good master.

Heart

When the Earth diverted to 23 degrees from its road, the heart also diverted at an angle of 23 degrees then. This is the reason for its location: a little to the left, and not in the middle. One day, when the Earth comes back to its initial state, the heart will come exactly at the middle, as it was with the original man.

Contemporary physiologists have a special notion about the heart. They consider it to be something like a pump, and due to its contractions and relaxes blood moves all over the body. This is partly true, but actually heart not only makes blood move. The reason for the blood movement is a special vital power, which comes as a flow into organism and makes heart cells pulse. This power has its own regulator in the brain. Hence heart cells are Rational creatures with great intelligence. After the brain cells, heart cells come next if we speak about intelligence.

Contractions and relaxations of heart happen thanks to electricity, which comes down from a special zone. Brain regulates the zone of the heart. Many people die untimely, because that electrical current, which comes from outside, is interrupted. Just as wheels move by a dynamic force, the heart is controlled by a cosmic force of the Universe. Thanks to that force, the heart contracts and relaxes, i.e. constant tides occur. At each contraction and relaxation of the heart, the blood is received and sent all over the body.

Actually, the heart, as a physical organ, and has no a power to push the arterial blood in the body. The reason for the pulse of the heart is due to the cosmic electricity and magnetism. They bear life. When the harmony between these powers is destroyed, the function of the human heart is also destroyed.

Blood is a conductor of human life. By its increasing or decreasing, life is prolonged or shortened. Blood has two major components: one - liquid plasma, and the other – of red and white corpuscles and some others. Blood bears oxygen, which is needed for life, to the organism. It takes the carbon dioxide, which has formed in the body. It is a poison and through the venous blood, it takes it out. This purification happens during all the time. When our thoughts are unclean, carbon dioxide increases. When our thoughts are clean oxygen increases and carbon decreases. When our heart is clean, oxygen increases, and carbon decreases. If your deeds are right, oxygen also increases, and carbon decreases. Right deeds increase oxygen in the body. Right feelings increase oxygen in the heart and right thoughts increase oxygen in the human mind. If you destroy the plasma of your blood, in your heart, by the feelings, if you destroy the plasma of your blood, in your body, by your deeds, I ask, who can help you? You will begin to sniff.

Heart is the pulse of the whole Cosmos. In higher mathematics, there are calculations, which we do not know. There are certain tables, in which calculations, concerning the pulsing of all people's hearts, are made. There are no two people, who have the same heartbeat. Some people's hearts make 10 beats and a break occurs. Other people's hearts make 20 beats and then a break, third people's hearts make a break after 30 beats; fourth people's hearts – after 100 beats, etc. Do you know for what these break are? This is a connection to other worlds. Hence, according to the ratio of the rhythm, that interval shows to which worlds you are connected – to the Milky Way or other constellations. At that moment, these worlds introduce various virtues into your soul.

As for the heart beat, it is noticed that during the first 12 hours of the day, the heart beats faster and with a couple of beats more than the normal heartbeat. During these 12 hours, the heart is in an ascending state. During the second 12 hours of the day, i.e. during the second half of the day, the heart beats decrease and the heart is in a descending state. The same is noticed in the course of months and years. The first 14 days, the heart is in an ascending state; the second 14 days, the heart is in a descending state. The first half of the year, the heart is in an ascending state; the second half of the year, the heart is in a descending state. It is important for everyone to know when his heart is in an ascending state and when it is in a descending state.

When man lives normally, after the law of Love, his pulse is normal. If he breaks that law, his pulse changes. All negative states, through which man passes – doubt, suspicion, discouragement, disbelief, influence the pulse. If one does not know that, he alone causes misfortunes to himself. Because of his negative thoughts and feelings, one changes the run of the cosmic pulse – a bearer of God's blessing.

The pulse does not beat well, when you eat hard to digest food or if you are in a trouble. The brain and stomach systems are not in good shape then. This continues till the right relation between the brain, lungs and stomach restores. After that, pulse will also regulate. When a disharmonious feeling occurs in us, e.g. hatred, the pulse again will not beat normally.

From time to time man shall measure the pulse of his heart and see if its rhythmic or not. If his pulse is not rhythmic, this shows that there is something wrong with his feelings.

The right thought never upsets nerves. Do not mix the heart functions with the ones of the brain. The task of the heart is to send unclean blood into the lungs in order it to be purified and to be sent all over the body as arterial blood. Heart does not purify only blood, but feelings, too.

Man has three hearts: one of them is in the pit of the stomach, the other

– between lungs and the third one – at the back of the head. When these three hearts function normally, when heart moves blood normally, man is in a normal state.

Digestive System

One, who has a healthy and normal digestive system, he is joyful, cheerful, and diligent. If you meet somebody with a dry face, yellowish, unwilling to work, you shall know that his digestive system is in bad shape. He cannot work; he takes a gloomy, pessimistic view of things; he has no faith in life. In order not to fall in such a condition, keep your digestive system in good shape. The well-being of the physical world, the first step of life, depends on it.

The brain and stomach are two poles of life. If you have a headache, you shall know that your stomach is a mess, too. If you have a stomach-ache, you shall know that your head is also in bad condition.

When pores are opened, the stomach functions well, normally. Pores are channels, through which energies of Nature find their way to the organism. A healthy and normal digestive system ensures a normal brain system and thanks to that – a normal respiratory system.

Hell is in man's intestines. That is why when one shall undergo a treatment, at first he shall clean his stomach and his intestines.

The more stomach works, the less brain works and vice versa.

It is not enough only gastric juices to be generated during digestion, but they have to be normally oxidized, in order they to give pure red colour to the blood.

Pure blood contains in itself all vital elements, as well as kinetic and potential energy, which are the reason for forming of the mind. During circulation, there is also back flowing of blood, which may return to man's spiritual body. Circulation is not only a physical process, but also a spiritual one. Under a physical process we understand only that, which is visible and may be tested. However, there are things which are not visible for the naked eye and cannot be tested.

When digestion is not proper, sludge remain in the body, and then the serum, in which bacilli multiply, is generated. This is the first phase, and the dung, left by the microbes, start the second phase.

Liver

Liver is a great factor in the human body. If the liver stops functioning, man departs this life. At the present structure, the liver solves everything. If it is upset, man becomes indisposed, dark; he is a pessimist; he cannot talk carefully; he hates; he is angry; he can commit a murder and all this comes out of the liver.

If the liver of somebody upsets, negative and unpleasant thoughts pass through his mind. The upset of the liver promotes cruelty in man. The liver is connected to the lower feelings. Knowing this, man shall sacredly keep his health, which was given to him by God.

Man lives with four bodies: physical, astral, mental and causal. Each body performs a specific service and is composed of a specific matter, and each organ of the physical body is connected to the astral, i.e. with the world of feelings. It regulates man's lower feelings, absorbs poisons in the the organism and transforms them. If it upsets, poisons go all over the organism and man dies. There is a close relation between the liver and the gall. If the relation is broken, life is in danger. As the liver is connected to creatures from the lower astral life, they start influencing man and whisper pessimistic philosophy to him or make him commit suicide. These creatures are strong, but not organized. As they do not understand life, they are ready to kill everyone, who blocks their way. If you go into a painful state of the soul, you shall know that you are in the sphere of the unorganized matter. Saints have good liver and organized supreme feelings. The organized liver is the best servant of the heart. The upset of the liver causes various diseases. Neurasthenia is due also to an upset of the liver. One, who is not ready to oblige people, does not communication with God, he is ill, his liver is upset. When you get angry, turn to God with a request to give you more knowledge and light in order to get your liver in good shape. If you cannot stand people, if your things do not go well, if you cannot study, your liver is guilty. Its upset affects the brain abilities and man's feelings, as well as his spiritual manifestations. The lower feelings influence the liver like termites, which eat everything. One, who has organized his feelings and thoughts, he has also organized his liver. He is ready to become reconciled with all people. You see how important the liver is for everybody. He is related even to faith. To have faith in God means to have an organized liver, to have an organized mind, heart and soul. Under "faith in God", it is understood one Divine state, at which man feels himself strong enough to achieve everything he wants. Faith is a power, through which everything is achieved. It is useful for organizing the liver.

The good or bad condition of the liver affects also man's feelings, and feelings influence the state of health of the liver.

The insult, which you experience, affects the liver as a bitter feeling, with which you cannot easily cope. If you see that one's face becomes yellow or red, look for the reason in the liver.

If the liver gets ill, it is hard for healing; it is connected to man's cerebellum.

The liver is needed, but when it expands too much, misfortunes occur. If it becomes small, it will be also bad. The liver shall function in order to create the gall.

Hairs

Hairs serve for regulation of the energies in the human organism. Each hair is a centre of a dynamic power, which helps for the distribution of the blood along the surface of the body. The hairs are so much necessary to man as plants to the Earth.

Hairs, which Nature has given to man, are nothing else than antennas, through which he can communicate not only with the remote places on the Earth, but also with the other planets. Hence, through his hairs man can perceive the vibrations of the Sun, the Moon, Mars, Venus, Jupiter and communicate with them. All hairs do not perceive equally the vibrations like man's eyes, which do not perceive equally the light. One of the eyes perceives better than the other. The fingers have also different perceptive ability. The whole man's body is a sum of lots of antennas. In this respect, he is a knot, of which lots of antennas – perceivers of lots of thoughts, feelings and desires - come out.

It is known that plants and trees keep the moisture in the soil. The trees are pumps, which draw out the moisture to the surface of the earth. Hence, the role of the hairs for the human organism is the same as the role of the trees for the soil. They regulate the moisture in man's body.

You have 250 thousand of hairs only on your head – the most beautiful adornment. Some of them are put on the centre of faith, others on the centre of conscience, third ones perceive the waves of justice, charity, etc. These hairs perform something great. To think means to perceive. Do not think that somebody can create a thought only by himself. You shall attract the thought from creatures, which stand a lot higher than you – I am talking about harmonious thoughts. In order you to have noble feelings, you shall attract the feelings of higher creatures.

All hairs on the head are not made in one and the same way. Each hair differs, if only insignificantly, by thickness, colour, and quality. Hairs are not only yours, but of thousands of generations before you. You have at your disposal the radio of the old people. The head is a radio. Hairs are antennas. When the radio is well tuned, there is no hissing and thoughts are delivered clearly.

Each hair is an antenna. Each hair is a conductor of the light. You do not know what relation hairs have to the external powers of Nature. That is why they shall be always kept in good order. In order powers to pass normally through them, run your fingers frequently through them. When you are nervous or in bad spirits, wet your hair a little and smooth it again by fingers or a comb.

It is well for a woman to have long hair.

If you have become too mild or if your will has weakened, it is well to cut your hair as a solder to the skin. If you have become too rough, let your hair grow.

Your hair shall be always smoothly combed. I recommend to one, who are nervous, to mess his hair up before going to bed in the evening, to disarrange it and after that to run his fingers through it for several times and go to bed then and comb it well in the morning.

Senses

The original man, created in the image of God, had 12 senses at his disposal. In the process of involution, he gradually lost his senses, while he remained with 5 senses as the present man. That is why the ratio between his present knowledge compared to the past one is 5:12.

After the sense of touch, the sense of taste, smell, hearing and finally eyesight appeared. Five senses – five cultures. This is the history of the human soul by now. There are more senses, which man shall develop. His ear and eye will change. They will obtain a more perfect form than the present one. After 3 thousand years, there will be an enormous difference between the man of that time and the man of the present. The present man will look like a savage to the future man.

Man's eye is created at the end. It is of the highest origin. All more eminent clairvoyants, all adepts and teachers read and study by the eye.

The powers, through which human intelligence and wisdom manifest, have created the nose and ears. The powers, the energies, through which love manifests, have created the mouth. Truth has created the eyes, eyebrows and eyelids. Rationality has created the forehead.

The matter, of which the eyes are made, is prepared at another place, and it is only projected on the Earth. If it happens man to damage any of his organs, it cannot be repaired, because the parts of this organ are not here and cannot be fixed and hence the organ cannot be fixed, too. The nervous system, which rules the mental and nervous temper, penetrate through the whole body, transfers the blood through the entire body. Its organs are the road messages for man. The second thing is man's lungs, which are connected to the dynamic powers, to the electricity and magnetism. They deal with the air, with prana, which is perceived by the lungs and is delivered to the blood, which is purified through prana and is transferred along the entire body to the most remote nourishing centres.

The sanguine (gaseous) temper has formed in this way. In order man to be healthy, his lungs shall be well developed. If the mind is better developed than the heart, shoulders are wide and straight. If the feelings are more developed, shoulders are rounded.

According to me, one is beautiful if he has healthy eyes, ears and a healthy mouth. Eyes are connected to the brain, the ears – to the heart, to the sympathetic nervous system, and the mouth – to the stomach and the liver.

The state of the lungs depends on the structure of the nose – its size and width. In addition, the form of the nose is responsible for the form of the lungs, but in a reverse position.

What is the nose? It is a place of electricity and magnetism. It is a peak, where the energies of Nature are stored. Bad thoughts influence the nose and therefore the respiratory system. If it does not work well, the stomach system suffers. As a result of that the balance between the mental and sympathetic nervous systems is destroyed.

Sometimes it is well man to put his finger at the beginning of the nose, between the eyes. In this way one may concentrate. Those, who are distracted, shall put a finger on the top of the nose, in order to think. You will concentrate and gather your thoughts a little. You shall put gently your finger either between the eyebrows, at the beginning of the nose or on the top of it. The arms are an extremely mighty power, two poles. The positive power is in the right arm, and in the left arm - the negative power.

All painful states are reflected in people's eyes. There circles cross, by which the right flows in the eyes are interrupted.

The eye is a living Divine form, in which it is written how the whole Cosmos, the whole solar system and finally the life are structured.

There is not a more perfect organ than the eye. The little light, which you perceive, is so transformed that it illuminates the whole body. And this light, when it goes out, it illuminates the whole world.

Those, who have brown eyes, need warmth. They shall wash their feet with warm water every evening. Those, who have blue eyes, need moisture; when arms and feet begin to get cold, they shall drink 3 or 4 cups of hot water. These are external methods, through which man shall help himself. For people with brown eyes, warm baths, with a temperature from 35 °C to 41 °C, are recommended. Internal peace and calmness is recommended for people with blue and grey eyes. Their minds shall be busy, but not with great, unsolvable matters, but with ones, which are a prerequisite for their development. When Nature painted people's eyes in various colours – brown, blue, black, it wanted to show man what he is missing. Man with brown eyes is affectionate, he is easily attracted. One, who has blue eyes, is considered to be an idealist. He likes to think of higher matters, to be in the clouds. Those, who have brown eyes, if they eat meat, shall eat mainly lamb meat. Those, who have blue eyes, shall eat more fish.

Sensibility, which we have in fingers, depends very much on the small papillae. Our delicateness also depends on them. These papillae shall not be damaged. They shall not be put under sudden changes in temperatures.

The four fingers of the arm are connected to the angles, seraphim, cherubim and archangels. The thumb is connected directly to the Divine world. Knowing this, pet them frequently. Connect yourselves to those powers, to which the arm is connected. Never hide your thumb between the other fingers. Through fingers, one gets in contact to the Spiritual world, in which Rational creatures, which are always ready to help, live. It is a misfortune if any of the fingers, especially the thumb, is affected. The human arm is beautiful. The development of the mind and the heart depend on it.

Thumb is connected to the face. It is the Divine in man. The thumb belongs to the nobleness, honour, dignity. The middle finger sees good and bad in everything. It belongs to justice and logic. It is very strict.

Elegance of life is connected to the solar finger (the nameless one). The small finger belongs to the application, to the calculations, to the attitude to the others.

The state of health belongs to the thumb. It is the Divine and it shall be always on the top. You shall not hide it.

If the mind, the heart and the will function normally, then the finger will also move well. If the mind functions normally, the thumb of the right hand will also move normally. If the heart functions normally, then the thumb of the left hand will move normally. If both thumbs move normally, this means that the will is right. When man gets mentally ill, this influences the thumb and the other fingers.

Finer Bodies

The virgin Divine Spirit came down in a circular wave across seven fields, across seven worlds, during the Saturn period to the mental world and formed man's mental body. During the second period – the solar one – the Spirit came down to the astral world and formed the body of desires. During the third period – the Moon one – the Spirit came down to the ether sphere of the physical world and formed the ether casing of the body. During the fourth period – the Earth one – the Spirit came down to the lower sphere of the physical world and formed the physical body. During the first period, when the Divine Spirit worked and created man in the image of God, man was worriless. During the second period he began to fall. During the third period, he came to complete degradation, and during the fourth period – the Earth one, which is the lowest period of coming down – the degradation reached its utmost limit. Man came down and sank in the matter, in order to dress in all casings, more and denser, from where his entrance and dressing in higher forms begins. Partial coming down and climbing happen along a wave-like line happens during each period. The final movement will be ascending.

The most familiar of all bodies is the physical one, which consists of three casings. One of them is of ether and comes out of the physical body up to 12 cm. Physical powers with electricity and magnetism pass through it. We dress our physical bodies with warm or thin clothes, in order to protect it against cold or hot weather. The ether casing is also a health clothing of the physical body, which protects it against external influences. The ether casing is related to another one- the astral, which rules lusts. It protects man, for example from anger, from his desire for revenge, etc. The astral casing is related to the astral world, called subconscious.

One day, when people develop their sixth sense, they will see that there is a casing round man's body. While this casing exists, man is healthy, because it regulates the warmth of his organism. Sometimes, under the influence of bad life, that magnetic casing round man's body breaks and the external influences penetrate into it, causing lots of diseases. That magnetic clothing wraps up the stomach, lungs, all internal organs in man's body, as well as its cells.

While he is on the Earth, man works mainly by his physical body – the most suitable instrument for the Earth. However, he thinks, feels, looks for the reasons and consequences of things. By what does man think? By his mental body. By what does man feel? By his astral body. By what does he find the reasons and consequences of things? By his causal body. Physical body is not equally developed with all people. The same is valid for the rest bodies in man. This shows that man is in front of a big and great work – development of all his components to perfection.

Through feelings, man is connected to the astral world, i.e. to his astral body, called also "spiritual body". The astral body consists of two spheres: lower and higher, depending on the feelings, which also can be higher or lower. The astral world is liquid like water. There creatures live like fish in water.

Man shall obey the law of sequence in the three worlds. In the physical world, he shall know how to feed, how to breathe, how to drink water and how to perceive light. He shall have well organized physical body. If he enters in the spiritual world, he shall have a well organized astral body. For the mental world, he shall have a well organized mental body. One, who has developed his three bodies, he may be called a wise man. Man's physical body is as important as his astral and mental bodies.

Man lives on the Earth both with his mental and his causal bodies; they are connected to higher than the physical and astral worlds. Hence, man lives with four bodies: physical, astral, mental and causal. Each body has a special service. Each body is composed of a specific matter. Each organ of the physical body is connected to one of the four worlds. The liver, for example, is connected to the astral one, i.e. to the spiritual world or to the world of feelings. It regulates man's lower feelings. It absorbs the poisons in the organism and transforms them. If it gets upset, the poisons go all over the body and man dies.

The physical body has its physiology and anatomy. The same is with the astral, mental and causal bodies. The physiology and anatomy of the higher bodies are similar to those of the physical body.

After each period of seven years, man begins a new phase – development of a new body. There are seven bodies of the kind. In the spiritual development, there are three more bodies, and there are two more at the most advanced. Hence, totally 12 bodies may develop in man.

In the front part of the brain, there is a special type of white brain threads, through which the activity of human conscious manifests. The conscious is related to the doppelganger, the so called ether body of man or a mediator of powers in Nature. Man's physical body lives thanks to his doppelganger. Hence, if the relations between the doppelganger and the physical body are normal, harmonious, man will always be healthy. If these relations are not harmonious, lots of painful states arise in man. And vice versa – when any of the organs of the physical body gets ill, the harmony between the doppelganger and the physical body breaks. That is why, in order you to recover from a disease, your first work shall be directed to restoration of the normal relations between your spiritual body and the physical one.

When you deal with spiritual works, excessive energies accumulate and certain dangerous states are caused. The spiritual person becomes extremely sensitive. Everything affects him. His ether doppelganger prolongs more outwardly. His astral body expands and he begins to complain that he cannot bear people's influence.

You shall understand the law – how to gather into yourselves. When you learn the law, you will not let the doppelganger go out. There, where the influences are harmonious, you may expand as much as you want, but if you come upon unfavourable conditions of life, you shall gather.

When the doppelganger goes out of man, the latter lives almost like an animal: he eats, drinks and thinks about nothing. By knowing that, you shall be careful and avoid startling each other, especially while you are sleeping. When man sleeps, his doppelganger comes out of him and goes to the space. During that time the doppelganger is connected to the body only by one thread. If you awake somabody and startle him suddenly, his doppelganger does not manage to come back to the body and as a result of this it entangles with other doppelgangers in the space. If one does not know how to untwist his doppelganger, he goes crazy.

According to occultism, each of man's bodies is a certain magnitude. The physical body is one magnitude, the astral body – a second one, the mental body – a third one, and the causal body – a fourth one. Each of these bodies has its specific energies. You shall understand these energies, to be able to transform them and turn them from one world into another.

The bodies are three-dimensional, but the soul cannot be three-dimensional. The world of feelings is four-dimensional. The mental world is five-dimensional, and the causal world is six-dimensional. The soul is from the seven-dimensional world. The other world, which comes after this world, is exactly the same as our world is for the animals. The spirit is from the tenth dimension.

Man's soul has its special body, with which he can ascend. This body is so plastic and so well made, that it may become small and big. Exactly that body builds the physical body and all other man's bodies, about which it is known that they are seven, but I think that they are twelve. What I speak to you today, one they will be checked by you, and you will see that it was true.

The physical body gives us the rough material and serves as scaffolding for building of the spiritual body, with which we will materialize and dematerialize, when we go to the spiritual world. If the soul in the physical body has not managed to build a spiritual body, after the death it remains poor like an orphan child and cannot manifest itself, because there is no a source of power for it.

The human body is a prison, in which the soul stays temporarily.

The spirit, the soul and the mind do not die. The soul is a principle, the

33

spirit is a principle and the mind is a principle. The physical body is a result of the human mind. The mind may make for itself whatever body it likes.

Do not try to win over the flesh in yourselves. The spiritual in man cannot develop without flesh. It is like a pad in the plant, on which the grafting is realized. There is a struggle between the flesh and the spirit, which continues till the spirit, i.e. the graft, fixes well on the pad and starts developing normally by itself. When the juices from the pad start moving normally upwards to the graft, and those from the graft start moving normally downwards to the pad, life develops normally. Then we say that the struggle between the flesh and the spirit is over. This is also called transformation of energies. Each man shall know that law and apply it in his life. In order man to be able to apply correctly that law, he shall pray.

Energies

Each physic energy is a manifestation of God.

The energy of our physical, mental and moral life comes from the Sun. I do not speak about the physical sun, about the disk, which we can see, but about the other Sun, which is invisible (behind the physical one). It produces all invisible results.

Living creatures are doors, conductors of energies. The highest energies pass through man – the highest form.

There is a certain energy, which comes down from the Sun and is invisible. When this energy comes to the Earth, the female principle turns this energy and light is born. Light was born by the woman on the Earth. Energy has come from the Sun through the man. Energy will come through your brain, through your head. This energy transforms through your stomach brains (the solar plexus) and life begins to function.

The more intensive is energy, contained in our organisms, the more favourable it is. The less intensive is the energy, the more harmful it is.

Many of the creatures, which live in the physical world, are in a low development phase, as a result of which they draw power from those creatures, which are at a higher level than them. If you get on their road, they will by no means draw from you and you will feel powerless. In order you to restore the spent power, you shall contact the sublime world and draw energy from there. Whatever you do, you cannot get rid of the influence of the lower world. Hence, at one place they will draw from you, at another place you will draw. In other words, while man is connected to the Earth, he always loses his energies. When he contacts the Sun, he draws from its energies and renovates himself.

There are 700-800 million of separate nerves in our bodies, through which we perceive energies from Nature. Do you know that millions of creatures have worked for these wires?

In each human cell, there is so much energy that it can displace the axis of the Earth at 1 meter away from its path. What power would man have been, if all cells were in harmony! Today people use their power more for destruction than for building. If the power of the mind is used for creative work and building, what enormous results would be achieved!

Man draws his vital powers from a couple of sources: food, air, water and light. He also draws energies from the mind, feelings, and his deeds.

Man can also draw energy for the maintenance of his organism from the light, if he knows its laws; from the life, if he understands it, and from the love, if he aims at it. These are three sources, from which man can draw power, life, and health.

There shall be no an excess of energy in the organism, but exactly so much as it is needed. Excessive energy shall be returned to Nature.

Man is a equilateral triangle with a common centre, to which all of his energies are directed. In other words, man is a sum of energies, which aim at one centre. And vice versa – man is a sum of energies, which go out of a common centre and disperse in different directions.

What is the physical body? The physical body is a conductor, i.e. a great installation of the powers in Nature. Through this installation, two types of natural powers pass: positive and negative electricity, positive and negative magnetism. For the present, our bodies are not physically toned: one of us are positive, and others – negative, i.e. some people have more positive electricity in themselves, and others – more negative electricity.

Only the negative energies create. If you are a clairvoyant, you will see that the light appears only on the negative pole. When they say about somebody that he is attractive, it means that he has negative energy in himself – this is magnetism. Such a person has something for giving to and something for taking from people.

Magnetism and electricity are powers, which come from God (I do not speak about the mechanical powers). When these two powers from God come down, magnetism goes into the heart, and electricity – into the mind and thanks to them man can move lots of obstacles away from his path.

Magnetism is a power, which promotes the development of the Universe and the development of all living creatures. The movement of the Moon round the Earth, of the Earth round the Sun, of the Sun round other suns – all that is due to magnetism. Magnetism maintains the harmony in Life, in the entire Universe. If it flaws away, life cannot manifest itself. If one loses his magnetism, he becomes dissatisfied, dark, and everything looks ugly and dark to him. One, who has less magnetism, he will be always cold even if he is at a warm place. Magnetism gives attractiveness and warmth to man.

Energies of magnetism go along curve lines, which wind like a spiral and produce warmth. To a great extent, our heath is due to the magnetic energies, which flow in the organism. The electrical energies go mostly along straight lines. Man shall understand the laws, in order to be able to cope with the excessive amount of electricity and magnetism in his body. Electricity and magnetism are powers, which function from outside. These powers polarize each other, but man shall know the laws, after which they function, in order to be able to transform them intentionally.

For the present, the vital energy, which is contained in Nature, as well as in all elements, is not found yet. It is called prana by the Hindus or vital electricity. Such energies are contained in our organisms in the elements hydrogen and oxygen, but are not hydrogen and oxygen; the latter are only bearers of these energies.

Prana has various states: it is physical, heart, mind or mental. Without prana, a thought cannot be formed; without prana, feelings cannot appear and without prana, will cannot function. Prana is the reason for creation and manifestation of thoughts, feelings and man's deeds. This does not mean that all people have equal thoughts and feelings. Each man, in accordance with his development, will accept what he needs and will manifest what he can.

Prana is needed for the human organism. Man's health depends on it. That is why it is recommended people to go out early in the morning in order to take in a larger quantity of prana. After that they have to process energy, which they have taken in and use it wisely. If you do not use it, it will cause you troubles.

The Hindus have scientific theories for the formation of prana in man's organism. According to them, each man, who can wisely and correctly use prana, he can get rid of all diseases: in the stomach, lungs, eyes, etc.

At the beginning of spring there is more prana and organisms take it in more. During the summer, the warmth is more, but not prana. There are certain features, after which it can be guessed when there is more prana accumulated in Nature.

The mountains are warehouses of energies, which help people to transform their states.

Special creatures come down from extremely high worlds and process our mental energy, in order it to become suitable for people's minds. Do not think that human brain needs the same energy, which is needed by the stomach. The energy, at which the stomach functions, is different. The same concerns the lungs and brain.

In order the form of a noble, sublime idea to be generated in the brain, a specific energy is needed. That energy involves only the top part of the forehead. The bottom part of the forehead may understand another idea.

Man shall understand the laws, after which the living electricity and the living magnetism function, the so called by the Hindus prana. The spinal cord is the main perceiver and transmitter of prana. First prana goes to the cerebellum, and from there – to the cerebrum. If any blockage occurs in the cerebellum, prana cannot continue its path to the cerebrum, as a result of which disharmony establishes in it. That disharmony is delivered to the entire organism.

At the negative pole are the feelings, at the positive – the thoughts. The brain is positive, and the sympathetic nervous system - negative. In the left side of the human body, the energy goes downwards to the left leg and then, along the right leg and along the right side, goes upwards. There is such an electromagnetic flow around each organ. For example, positive energy passes along the right eyebrow. It turns from there and goes under the right eye and turns into negative energy. It goes up from there over the left eye and it is again positive there. After that it goes down under the same eye as a negative energy. In this way, during its movement, that energy forms something like the figure of eight. In the point between the eyebrows or in the root of the nose, there is a rational centre, which regulates these flows round the eyes.

The energies in the human brain are divided into 3 major spheres: the first sphere is behind the ears, where the lower energies function. That sphere can be compared to man's hell. The second sphere involves the energies, which function in the sphere of the forehead – the human life. The third sphere involves the energies in the top part of the brain, where the higher moral feelings function. That sphere can be compared to the paradise in man. Hence, when one counteracts his moral feelings, the energy from that sphere goes down, behind the ears, in hell. In order this not to happen, one shall let his good desires free, and not block them.

You know from physics that the energy from the positive pole goes to the negative one. Do you know through what path the positive energy passes? It usually goes out of the right hemisphere of the brain, goes along its surface, passes under the left hemisphere, then turns over it and goes back under the right hemisphere. Here, in the negative pole, light is generated. Hence, the thoughts come from the right hemisphere, pass through the left one and as a result of that light are produced in the consciousness.

There is one Moon flow and one solar flow. The solar flow comes from the right side of the brain, goes into the left part and goes out of the back part of tail, down. This is the lowest man's brain. The other flow passes from the left side and goes to the right part. We have the same flow through the nostrils during breathing.

One of the flows is of the mind, and the other - of the heart. They both form a figure of eight.

The energy of the right half of the brain goes to the left. That is why contemporary people think only with the left part of their brains. This is the reason for the asymmetry of man's face. If we take a careful look at the human face, we see that both sides (the left and the right) are not equally developed. That difference is also noticed in the eyes, in the ears, in the mouth, in the arms, in the entire body.

If more energy gathers in the right hemisphere, man becomes nervous, he cannot stand still. If more energy gathers in the left hemisphere, man becomes active.

Man shall work with both sides of his brain (left and right) in order to distribute equally his energies.

Contemporary people do not obey that law, as a result of which they suffer of another physiological defect, and namely: the blood is not distributed equally along all organs of their bodies. In the healthy organism the blood is distributed equally along all organs of its body. Man's thoughts shall also penetrate through all cells of the organism. One can be healthy only in this way.

If you touch the hand of a healthy man, you will notice that one of its sides is warm, the other is cold; one of the arms is warm, the other – cold; half of the head is warm, the other half - cold.

It is not like that with somebody, who is ill. The flows in him are changing: they are either warm, or cold. This is so, because of the caused imbalance of the powers in his organism. For the purposes of treatment, one shall restore the internal balance of his powers. If this is achieved, he recovers.

There are two poles in man as on the Earth there are two poles (north and south), which are a warehouse of energy.

Your mind will produce a cold flow in you, the heart will produce a warm flow and from these two flows, a rotation, a movement is established. This movement bears the normal life – this is the internal circulation in man. The contradiction is the fact that sometimes the mind produces a larger quantity of coldness than the needed one, and sometimes heart develops more warmth than the needed one.

The higher man stands, the more light comes out of him. People say about such a man that he is magnetic; he influences the minds and the hearts of the surrounding people. In his presence, even the most excited and nervous man calms down. Magnetism is a flow, which flows freely and independently out of man. This flow shall not be interrupted. Who can interrupt the magnetic flow in man? Somebody, who is bad and evil.

How can we guess if we have magnetism? If you are in good spirits – you have magnetism. If you are not in good spirits, if you are nervous, you have not magnetism. Magnetism gives the good spirits.

The little children are the most magnetic persons. That is why we are so attracted by them.

Moisture regulates the influence of the electricity on the human organism. The electricity dries man, makes him thin and delicate. Sometimes it can dry him so much that his nerves may be thinned and unable to endure the surrounding environment. If magnetism takes an advantage, man gets fat a lot. If such man eats a little, he again gets fat.

When man is ready to quarrel with everybody, whom he meets, this shows that there is an excess of electricity in the right half of his brain. When man is in bad spirits, when he becomes pessimistic, this shows that there is an excess of electricity in the left half of his brain.

In the front part of the brain electricity functions, and the back one - magnetism. In this way namely the powers in man's organism balance and he thinks rightly and enjoys good health.

The excessive energy causes lots of diseases. When somebody, who is fat, gets ill, electricity shall be introduces into his organism, and magnetism – in one, who is dry. Dry people shall mix with stout ones, in order a right exchange to happen between them.

The brain system is a dynamo, an accumulator of electricity, and the sympathetic nervous system accumulates magnetism. Neurasthenics frequently feel creeping along their legs, along the backbone – these are molecules of electricity, or pinches – these are small explosions of electrical energy. When electricity prevails and has predominance in the organism, one exhausts and becomes dry. The sympathetic nervous system serves as an accumulator of the living magnetic power, which comes from the Sun. When the predominance of the magnetic power begins to restore, the following happens with the neurasthenics: they begin to feel pleasant warmth from below. In the normal organism, when electricity and magnetism unite, they generate pleasant warmth, harmony of the powers.

When there are two harmonious thoughts, one of them is positive; it is connected to the cold flows in Nature. The other thought is a bearer of negative energy; it is connected to the warm flows in Nature. While one moves between these two flows, he feels well and healthy. Cold flows form in one of his brain hemispheres then, and in the other – warm, magnetic flows. When the head gets hot, man gets into painful state. In order his health to be restored, split mind shall be caused in him, i.e. two different flows to be created in his brain. When this state is achieved, the blood begins to circulate normally and man feels healthy.

Can one be healthy, if he never washes his feet, hands, face, and body?

The pores of the human body shall be always opened - they shall never get blocked. Pores have a magnetic casing, which shall be kept. One day, when people develop the sixth sense, they will see that there is a casing round their bodies and while this casing exists, man is healthy, because it regulates the warmth of his organism. Once, under the influence of bad life, that casing broke and the external influences penetrated in him and caused lots of diseases. That magnetic clothing wraps up the stomach, lungs, all internal organs and the cells.

Man breathes also through his pores, but unconsciously. Pores perceive prana from the air and in this way renovate organism.

In one, who is healthy, flowing out of electricity and magnetism happens constantly; there is always one vibration. When this vibration is normal, streams come out of the pores of the body, which throw the whole sweat out. Such a man is pious. That is why the bodies of pious people is clean; cleaning happens during all the time with them; there is a throwing from inside to outside. Water does not clean them. The vibration in them cleans them and in this way pores are never blocked. People can be healthy only in this way.

The backbone is the tenderest place: the biggest shocks happen there. Magnetic living energy flows along the backbone.

There are two flows in man. One of them is from the navel upwards and comes into being in the head and the other from the navel downwards. The second flow leads to the centre of the Earth, and the first one – to the centre of the Sun. Finally, there is a third flow, which unites the first two flows. The third flow is called aura of man.

The second flow, i.e. the one, which leads to the centre of the Earth, includes all lower man's energies, which he has gained in his animal state. By studying the structure of human body, we will see that the first two flows involve two more flows in themselves. All these flows are united in another one. They can be noticed also in man's thinking and feelings.

Blood moves not only because of heart's rhythm, but also under the influence of the electricity in Nature. While heart is under the influence of the living electricity, it contracts and relaxes uniformly, by sending blood all over the body. If the heart is not under the influence of the natural electricity, no circulation is possible. Why? It is so, because the resistance, which arteries and veins cause to blood movement, is so big that the heart would not be able to move it. It can receive energy from nowhere. It receives that energy exactly from the natural electricity.

Hence, if you want your heart to be healthy, keep your brain, from where the electrical flows of Nature pass and the solar plexus, from where the magnetic flows pass, in good order. In order your brain to be in good order, you shall avoid controversial thoughts. In order to keep the solar plexus in order, never let negative thoughts into your heart.

The primary light is the one, which moves the blood. Our circulation has a rhythm, an impulse, which is due to that cosmic energy – the electricity. The electricity is a form of light. The light is an impulse of that primary cause of the world. It fills the entire space.

The duties of the heart do not include only sending of the blood all over the body. It is also a knot of the electrical energy, which is delivered to all cells by giving them a chance to participate in the whole organic life. The lungs and the liver are two transformers of energy – the lungs are transformers of man's mental energy, and that is why it directs the energy of the mind to the brain; the liver – of the sensual energies, by directing them to the sympathetic nervous system. Feelings cannot manifest themselves without a lung.

A special kind of energy is generated by each gland. If man cannot create in himself mental and spiritual energies, this shows that the relevant organs in him are not awake. Man shall work on himself, to come to the state of emanating fine energy, with which to perform a higher work. For example, it is known that love has three poles, connected to three different centres: love to God, this centre is in the top of the head; love to the fellow men, this centre is in the middle of the head; and finally, love to yourselves – this centre is in the cerebellum. The last love is the most rough, because of the energies, which are developed in man. Today people live with that love, as a result of which, they think only of themselves. The centre of the love toward God is the most important one. And if the Bulgarians have suffered so much, this is a result from the the fact that that gland with them, this centre of love toward God is weakly developed. This centre is most developed with the Slavs, they love God in contrast to the Bulgarians. If the Slavs lose that love toward God, they will lose everything, because one's love is due to that centre – love toward God.

Arms are a dynamo; both currents of a battery and it depends on you how you are going to put them in order to regulate your flows. If you hold your hands loosely, you will be always weak. If you want to be in contact to the rational powers in Nature, tighten your arms well. If you want to be in contact to an Earth flow, you shall stretch out your arms, legs, the muscles of the entire body just for a few seconds and you will regulate the flows in you right away.

The palm of the left hand is the negative side in man, through which mild, magnetic vibrations are delivered. The top part of the left hand is positive, i.e. electrical. It is the same with the right hand. Hence, there are two types of electricity and two types of magnetism in man. One of the types of electricity and magnetism flow out from the left hand, and the other type – from the right hand.

On the top side of the human hand, positive electricity gathers and that is why it is hairy. The bottom side of the hand is passive and negative electricity gathers on it.

Frequently, more energy gathers in the left or in the right side of the body. Special type of currents flow out from the left or from the right hand. One of the sides is negative, the other - positive.

No matter how you put your hands, there is always flowing out, but when you unite them, the energies of Nature are more wisely used. If man keeps his hands closed for a long time, blocking appears in him. It is better if hands come into contact to each other only through the top of the fingers. When man locks, i.e. closes his hands, this shows that he is blocked, that there is some embarrassment in his soul.

From fingers comes out such an energy, which cannot go out from the silver and gold. Such an energy cannot go out even from the light.

From the first finger – the thumb – the most powerful energy comes out. The rest fingers are like the rear.

Each finger of the human hand is connected to a certain centre or organ of the brain. Each organ is connected to specific powers. These powers are connected to rational spheres and worlds. It is enough man to raise one of his fingers in order to contact the relevant organ, through which energies from the rational world flow.

Through each finger so much energy shall pass as it is needed for the development of the person.

Hence, the fingers perceive the energy, which come from the sublime world. As everything in Nature is accurately defined, each finger, each hand shall take in so much energy as it is foreseen. If it takes in more than it is needed, Nature will make you pay. How you are going to give back the excessive energy, which you have taken in from Nature? Through disease, through crises, through hardships.

In the middle of human brain is the so called flying eye of the soul or the internal sun of man. If that sun does not shine in man, nothing comes out of him. It plays the role of a transformer in the human organism. When the external energy penetrates into the brain of man, that knot, or the eye of the soul, resends that energy along the entire organism. It has also other functions, besides transforming of the solar energy. There is also another transformer in the brain, which takes in the solar energy along the entire body. The state of health of the organism, as well as of the feelings, depends on the correct transforming of these energies. Hence, that eye is a transformer of the Divine energy in man and creates conditions for his manifestation.

So, I tell you, as to disciples, first you shall train yourselves to control your brain. Gather the energy from Nature and resend it to the solar plexus, heart, trachea, forehead, the back side of the head and after that take that energy around your body. Start making those magnetic showers, while a light magnetic aura round the body forms and then you will feel yourselves free.

If man eats much, a big part of the brain energies go to the stomach, and he reduces the function of the brain by that. The brain is an accumulator of electricity and magnetism – the moment it succeeds in gathering that energy, food goes to the stomach, where it is devoured; it turns out that it works only for the stomach. That is why, each of us shall know how much, what and when to eat.

Man shall study his states, as well as the energies of his brain, in order to be able to transform them correctly. When man is angry, grumpy or in bad spirits, he shall know that this angry state is due to an energy, gathered round the hears, in the back part of the head and this energy shall be well distributed and transformed in order and explosion not to happen. It may be used for work and it shall be used wisely.

The anger is an energy, which is not used in a right direction. Everybody has felt weakness, one demagnetization after anger.

The anger, melancholy and bad spirits – this is all excessive energy, which can be transformed by taking the hoe and dig for 10 or 15 minutes.

Each sorrow, each hardship comes from that excess, which stays in man unused. That is why you shall study the law of turning of energies. There are people, who know how to transform not only their own energies, but also the ones of his friends or of the community.

To transform the energies means lower energies to be transformed into higher energies.

When a large quantity of energies gathers in one or the other side of your brain, you can influence alone yourselves. For example, if the electricity is accumulated in the right hemisphere of the brain, you shall not stroke your head by your right hand, in order not to increase your state, but you shall stroke the right side of your head by your left hand. And vice versa. If you have an excess of electricity in the left side of your head, you shall stroke it by your right hand. At this experiment, you will notice that you calm down and that you state is changing. That is why, during the summer, when the sun is shining violently over your head, stroke your hair by both hands. You will take out the electricity from the brain through your hands and you will avoid a sun stroke in this way.

As the brain is connected to all parts of the body, the polarization in some of its centres reflects right away in the relevant organs of the body, which, in this way, take part in the accumulation of energy. By knowing this, you shall look for a way for transferring the excessive energy in your organism from one centre to another.

There is a centre behind the ears of people, in which gathers more energy than it is needed. He becomes irritated, grumpy, and is ready to quarrel with everybody. If he can transform this energy and use it for some work, he will easily get rid of the anger. It is a special type of electrical energy. Look for a way of coping with the excessive energy round your ears. Begin to saw woods or to dig. If you cannot do that, touch the top of your nose 4 or 5 times. It is important to find a way to transform the energy of anger into work.

Sin is due to the personal feelings in someone. Personal feelings are a special sort of cosmic energy, which, if not transformed and distributed between all centres of the brain, causes an explosion. Near to the personal feelings is the centre of conscience, through which they have to pass. You shall learn the law of transforming of energies and direct them from one brain centre to another. You shall work the way Nature works. It has a certain time and place for everything. When one understands life, man obeys all laws and rules of Nature.

You are focus, through which the solar energies pass, as well as the Earth ones. The solar energies pass through you from the morning till noon. They come from up and go down to the centre of the Earth. In the afternoons, the movement is vice versa – the energies from the centre of the Earth pass through your legs and go up to the Sun. Hence, if you do certain movements in the morning and in the evening, you will have different results. Generally, bad spirits appear in the afternoons with some people, because the flows of the earth pass through them then.

You shall know how to polarize and concentrate these powers. Do not stop them. If you stop them, you will block yourselves and you may create a total catastrophe in yourselves. Resend these powers upwards.

Each man obtains energy from the spiritual world. If it is not so, he would not be able to live in the physical world, where he is always sucked and poisoned.

The different elements introduce different energies in the organism. For example, the gold introduces one type of energy, the silver – another and the iron – a third type. Hence, people differ in accordance with the different types of matters and energies and the differences of their quantity.

I say: when the vibrations of two bodies are not equal, that body, the vibrations of which are stronger affects the one, the vibrations of which are weaker. If two bodies with equal vibrations meet, there is a complete harmony between them.

People are connected to each other by something invisible, which causes a certain influence on them. This is the reason for which people influence each other consciously or unconsciously. People emanate a specific, dynamic energy, which affects the others, too.

People are interconnected, as a result of which energy may pass from one man to another, as liquids are poured from one vessel into another, when they are connected.

One, who is healthy delivers energy, the other – takes it in.

Man's aura is a circle, which is with a different colour, different size and thickness. Man's aura determines his mentality. Is the aura visible? For some people it is visible, for others – it is invisible. There is a centre in the middle of the aura, from where energies flow out: the upper energies are connected to the mental abilities of man, and the bottom – to the energies of his feelings. The upper energies are the masters, and the lower ones – the servants.

Man's aura is a natural barrier. When it is so, nobody has the right to enter without permission in the aura of somebody else. When somebody approaches you, he shall stand at 50-70 cm away from you. If he breaks this distance, if he approaches you too much, he establishes a disharmony in the relations. That disharmony is due to an incorrect exchange between the energies of both persons. One, who is sensitive, feels that incorrectness in the exchange and he begins to suffer. When the master speaks to his disciples, they gather round him, approach their heads to each other, but there is no incorrect exchange. Why? Because the thoughts of everybody are directed toward one common object. However, if two people with two opposite ideas approach each other at a distance less than 50 cm, a clash occurs. Their auras entangle and incorrect exchange happens between them. When they start feeling such a disharmony, they immediately move away from each other. Do not cross that sacred barrier, which has been put by Nature.

The energy, which nature has, is mathematically defined. It has distributed that energy impartially between all living creatures. It is accurately defined for everybody what energy to consume and what energy to spend. This concerns also thoughts and desires and not only food. You love a spiritual person and you want to sit with him for hours, to enjoy his aura. This is a crime. You shall enjoy his aura exactly as much as it is necessary, and you shall not stay for days and hours. It is the same when you drink water without a break.

When two people become close, their astral bodies connect to each other and begin to go from one of them to the other and vice versa. If one of them gets ill, the other gets ill, too. If a woman loves his husband and he dies, the woman dies, too. If a man loves his wife too much and if she dies dies, he dies, too. This happens if they are too much bound.

The duties of the animals are to gather magnetism. While animals are in good health, people will also be in good health; when animals begin to suffer, people will also suffer. That is why we shall be friendly towards animals, in order to profit by the magnetic powers, which they store in themselves.

Due to cleaning of forests and killing of mammals, people come upon big sufferings, without being able to help themselves. They do not even know that the animals and plants are a reservoir of vital powers for the growth and development of man. By killing mammals, their vital energy disperses in the space. As people cannot link directly to the powers of nature, they deprive themselves exactly from those vital powers, which are perceived by the animals.

Man gets older, because no more energy inflows into his organism. In the organism of one, who is young there is constant inflow of energy from Nature; one, who is able to harmonize in himself the energies of inflow and outflow, he can become young again.

As man is rich in energy, he spends is promiscuously. He does not know that for each energy, which is given to him, Nature holds him responsible for that. It credits him in all cases, but it gives, it is written down in a notebook. One day man will pay for the incorrect and unwise spending of the energy. It is a Divine energy and it shall be spent wisely.

If ordinary life manifests in you and you walk bareheaded, and the sun shines, toward noon you will have a sunstroke by no means, because that Divine energy will pass through the earth, will change some vibrations and will make the brain hot. However, if there is conscious life in you, and you show love toward all living creatures, you will turn that energy into "akasha" and you will feel in yourselves great, pleasant Divine music and great excitement will float along your entire body and you will wish to deliver your energy to everybody. All this will be in you, if you have a conscious life.

When one has been ill for a while, he loses a part of his vital energy. Here is what man can do in this case. Let him catch by his two fingers the lobe of the ear from time to time and pull it lightly downwards. Then let him massage the swelling behind the ear and watches for the changes that occur in his organism. Make these experiments not only when you are ill, but also when you are in bad spirits.

What shall we do when we are in bad spirits or if we have any mental embarrassment? Catch your ear by right finger and begin to think. After 1-2 minutes you will cheer up, normal exchange between the mental energies and the heart ones will take place. Each stagnation of vital energies in your organism is due to incorrect circulation. This stagnation stops the mental function. By knowing this, think of the ears and nose as of sacred places – conditions for correct perception and delivering of energies.

DISEASES AND HEALTH

Diseases

There are no diseases in the Divine world. Man creates the diseases, and not God.

The law is the following: when the body suffers, it is for the welfare of the soul.

In order to be able to endure the vibrations of the spiritual world, contemporary people shall strengthen their nervous systems. Presently, the white race is gradually adapting to the spiritual world. Sufferings, which they experience, are a preparation for the invisible world, in order people to get into contact with creatures from the sublime worlds.

Diseases show the roads of your diversion from the great Divine world or the right thought.

Diseases, of which contemporary people suffer, are three types: physical, i.e. ones, which affect the body; of the heart, affecting the feelings; and mental. The diseases of the physical body are healed in one way, of the feelings – in another, and of the nerves – in a third way. Contemporary medicine has no methods, through which diseases could be definitely eliminated.

49

When I speak of the good side of diseases, this does not mean that man shall be ailing. In addition, diseases are not only physical. Each indisposition, each sorrow, anguish is a painful state, which affects the organism. In this sense, diseases are visible and invisible, or physical and psychic. It is important for one to find a way for coping with them wisely. No matter how clever man is, he is always dissatisfied; he always wants something.

Who is mentally diseased? One, who is dissatisfied, doubts, does not master his mind, heart and will.

When one is ill, he is in the sufferings of the flesh. By suffering, he studies the laws of life. Each illness shows that a virtue is broken. The pain in the eyes, head, chest, stomach, as well as in all the rest organs, shows that these organs are deprived of something. The moment they obtain what they lack, the state of health will restore.

The disease is a consequence. While they live in ordinary conditions, people use the results of the past.

How perfection is achieved? Through sufferings. Then man goes down to the dense matter to study. If he does not suffer, he has no future. The sorrow is a raw material, which shall be processed. When it is processed, man climbs up towards joy. God, our Father, wants our perfection. He wants us to go to school and study. God's wish is we to study. It has to become our wish, too. God's wish is we to become perfect. It has to become our wish, too.

Suffering is the best thing on the Earth. There is no suffering, where there is no God. The good things of life come through suffering. If it could be without suffering, Jesus would have saved the world without suffering. One is great if he consciously bears the suffering. We, with our lack of understanding, cause sufferings to ourselves. The smallest unclean thought has the power to destroy the harmony of your life. The smallest unclean feeling and desire breaks the cleanness of your life.

When we understand the deep sense of the suffering, we will understand that this is a process, which forms our character.

Sufferings are a method, which Nature uses for softening one's rough feelings. When man suffers for a while, he gradually steps back and begins to think, to understand the poor and suffering people. Without sufferings, cruelness and roughness in man could not be softened.

Sufferings are roads, through which Nature throws away the unclean things from the human organism. Knowing this, thank for the sufferings, because without them, you would get poisoned.

There are sufferings in life, through which one shall pass by no means. They are foreseen by Nature. The rational sufferings are the needed load in a steamboat or in a boat, while they sail in seas and oceans. In order one boat or one steamboat to be able to sail, they shall, by no means, have a certain load at the bottom. That load balances the movement of the steamboat. Sufferings, therefore, are nothing else, but a ballast, which balances the powers in the human organism.

You always win in suffering. One, who does not suffer, is in stagnation. One, who suffers, grows.

The fixing of the world is God's work. Man's work is to fix his small world. How is he going to fix it? Man corrects himself through sufferings.

When God desires to make people know Him, He gives them sufferings.

What is the designation of diseases? When a living creature abuses with the powers, which are given to him, Nature sends him a disease, with which it limits him. Diseases, therefore, are nothing else, but a temporary limiting of one's freedom or of the freedom of the living creatures in general. The disposition, the limiting are nothing else, but painful states.

Contemporary people worry about small things. They do not know that diseases hide certain good things in themselves. Each disease is a task for someone. One, who solves his task, takes out the good, which is hidden in the disease, by himself. If they are angry about that, the good hides from them and more diseases reach them.

Diseases make people mild and delicate. People, who have suffered a lot, develop in themselves nobleness, delicateness, tenderness. People, who have suffered a little or never, are rude and cruel and I do not speak about the neurotics. These diseases are of another character. They have no organic origin. The neurotic diseases do not make people noble. On the contrary, they make them cruel.

The disease is live. When it enters in man and finds the relevant food, it stays to live in him. If it does not find food, it goes away. Therefore, remove all the conditions, which feed diseases and you will get rid of them.

Each indisposition introduces sediments, surpluses, inert matter in the organism, which have to be assimilated in a way, in order man not to get ill. That is why, Nature has admitted diseases as way of treatment. A disease is not a punishment, but an impulse, an encouraging reason, which makes man throw everything, which is unclean, away from himself.

Providence frequently sends to people big sufferings, in order to protect them against bigger ones.

If you want to recover, you shall come to the bottom of all sufferings. A suffering is a way of cleaning. You shall pass through the fire in order to clean yourselves. If you do not gain absolute cleanness, you cannot find what you are looking for. You can clean yourselves without sufferings, but only if you have been initially absolutely clean. If you are unclean, you will suffer.

After each disease, after each suffering, man gains a certain experience, which raises him. The more heavy the disease has been, the stronger he has become.

Influenza is cleaning for Christmas. Fever is cleaning for Easter. They both are cleanings.

Diseases are of educational importance for people. They strengthen the organism and prolong his life. It is known that people, who have suffered during their childhood, have strengthened their organisms, have made them more endurable against diseases and sufferings.

Diseases are necessary. They freshen. In order people to become milder, more sensitive, they shall suffer. The greatest people have suffered.

All diseases, sufferings, misfortunes in one's life are nothing else, but blessings, which God sends him and for which he has to be grateful.

When the thoughts, feelings and deeds of somebody are clean, he is not afraid, he does not worry. No matter what diseases come, he remains immune. Even if he gets ill, the disease will pass and go away, and will leave no traces. What is the reason about that? The clean blood is the reason. Therefore, in order you to endure diseases and sufferings, to cope easily with your contradictions, clean your thoughts, feelings and deeds. This is the so called internal purity. One, who has this purity in himself, his blood is clean. One's health, strength and good spirits depend on the purity of the blood.

You pay your duties through diseases. When you put in yourselves the desire to serve God, he pays for you and you recover in this way.

One, who always suffers, withstands diseases easier than one, who has never been ill.

There is more power in evil, and more mildness – in good. Power is united with mildness. If you manipulate, together with the good, the evil and if you decide to separate the good from the evil, you will develop an illness, which is incurable. If diseases are excluded from people's lives, they will come upon even worse evil than now when they suffer through diseases. Diseases make people milder. Lots of excessive energy has accumulated in man and it has to be regulated in a way.

When you come close to mild people, you feel certain pleasantness. This is due to the fact that mildness is pleasant, warm clothing, which wraps up such people. This warm and pleasant casing makes mild people immune to any kinds of diseases. Man's health depends on his mildness. When somebody loses his mildness, man begins to get dry and hard and he gets ill easily. Wherever he enters, whatever he looks at, he sees bad everywhere. Dissatisfaction is his companion.

Suffering is a spiritual process. It is the greatest thing in life and causes the biggest stirring of the powers in the human organism till they balance. People frequently experience big internal hardships, which are a result of blocked pores in the organism. Some big suffering shall come, in order these pores to be cleaned out. When you wash yourselves with water and soap, pores are cleaned only outsidedly, and their holes inside remain blocked. There are about seven million pores in man's body, which are major vents in human organism. When all pores are open, man is absolutely healthy, and this cleaning out happens only through internal washing, which we call 'sweating'.

Those microbes wedge in man, to which he is susceptible. They become partners with him and begin to benefit from his energies. Gradually he gets ill and becomes their victim.

We say that God lives in us, but we have rheumatism. And rheumatism remains. We say that God lives in us, but we have a tumor. And the tumor remains. God cannot live in a body, where there is ulcer or another disease. When the body gets absolutely clean and free of all diseases, the Spirit may enter and live there. At the present conditions, as long as your mind is not clear, as long as your legs, arms, head hurt, God is far away from you.

What is a disease? Unorganized matter, unorganized power, unorganized thought.

Diseases are your barometers. You can judge in accordance with them to where you have reached and what you lack. As long as you still pass through diseases, thank God and pray Him to help you to understand what you lack. For the present they are the negative side of your life. One day, when you overcome your diseases, you will come to the positive side of the life.

If somebody dislocates his leg or breaks it, this is a result from a bad thought or a bad deed. There is no a law, which will judge him for the thought, but he cannot get rid of the pain he feels. The doctor uses narcotic means, makes an operation and the sufferer does not feel pain, but after the operation, the pain increases. Nature is so clever that the punishment, which it wants to impose for the correction of one mistake, cannot be avoided, because it corrects it by that punishment. When I suffer, I understand that there is one creature out of me, which tells me: correct that mistake. If you do not want to correct it, I will correct it.

All painful states are not diseases. For example the cold and the fever are not diseases, but states of cleaning. The organism cleans through them from useless sediments and deposits. Tuberculosis, however, is a disease. There are psychic diseases, too. One, who judges himself, without correcting himself, he is ill.

Man needs only one thing – clean blood. The clean blood is able to cope with all diseases. It does not allow bacilli to develop in it. The vibrations of the clean blood are so powerful that all bacilli spring aside from it.

One, who is ill, has to give up something, but not air or food. He has to eat a little, but he has to choose his food. His illness is given to him exactly for education of his stomach. Give one, who is ill, a roasted apple, some walnuts and a small piece of baked bread. On the other day, instead of an apple, give him a roasted pear. The reason of all diseases, of all defects, of all misfortunes in life is spiritual, and not physical. If you want to be healthy, do not allow in your mind bad thoughts, negative feelings. The latter are parasites and shall not be left in your heads.

If you happen to have a furuncle, you shall know that the evil comes out through it. Each bad thought, bad feeling or deed manifests through rheumatism, furuncle or another disease.

Through cold and cough, man cleans his lungs and the entire respiratory systems from internal sediments.

The fever puts all unclean things to burning. When one of man's organs gets ill, his whole organism suffers. There is balance only when all organs are healthy and satisfied.

Diseases and man's working capacity depend on the vibrations of his brain.

Health restores through man's mind, and is maintained through man's feelings.

Diseases come periodically in the world. The more crimes with regard to love increase, the more diseases and anomalies in human life increase. If you apply the law of love in homes, communities and peoples, diseases will decrease right away. I do not speak about the human love, but about God's love, which raises man's spirit and solves all problems.

Health

Man's health depends on the following four things: the power of his soul, the goodness of his soul, the brightness of his mind and the mildness of his heart. In order one to gain these qualities, he shall have knowledge. Everybody has a soul, a heart and a mind, but not everybody has managed to develop such qualities in himself, which to make him healthy.

What is health? It is a capital, put in the bank. If every day you use the defined for that time capital, without depositing something, you will go bankrupt. If you deposit something every day, your capital will increase, i.e. your health will strengthen. Knowing this, do not wonder why, after being healthy, you fall ill. Lots of people use their capital, without depositing something in the bank and imperceptibly lose their health.

The truly healthy man is healthy in physical, mental and heart respect.

Health is related not only to the physical world, but also to the heart and mental ones. It is a result of the function of the higher laws, i.e. the laws of the Rational world. To be healthy means to be in harmony with the Original Reason of things, with your fellow men and with yourself.

Physical health is based exclusively on man's virtues. One, who is good, does not fall ill. If he begins to doubt good, he begins to fall ill. If one, who is ill, believes in good, he will recover by no means. When man sins, he goes out of the sphere of good and opens the door of sin in him. As long as he sins, he begins to fall ill. Death comes after the disease.

If man does not admit even one bad thought in his mind, even one bad feeling in his heart and even one bad deed in his will, no disease will catch him. Many bacilli will pass through him, but their poison will be enervated.

One, who wants to be in robust health, has to be connected to God by no means, to have a constant inflow of Divine energy.

You cannot be healthy, if you are not magnetic. When man feels that his nerves are exhausted, this means that he has demagnetized. Then he cannot hold the Divine thoughts, which only pass through him, without leaving anything. What will happen to a plant, if it does not accept the rainy drops and does not use them? You think that one, who is on the Earth, lives. As long as one is on the Earth, he is only tested. When the test is over, he is sent to another place.

Man may be physically healthy, be in good spirits to eat and drink well, but, spiritually, he may be not well, he may be not in the mood to do something good. By doing good, man spiritually feeds himself. If he is not in the mood to do good, this shows that he is spiritually ill. In order man to be spiritually well, this means that there shall be strong and stable feelings.

Absolutely healthy is one, in whose organism there are no sediments. One is healthy, if in his organism there is no decomposition, no decay. Everybody can be healthy or become healthy in one minute by exposing himself to special currents, which exist in Nature. Special rays exist in the Sun itself, special currents, which may revive man, only if he knows how and when to perceive these rays in order to benefit by them.

Health depends on man's conscious. Peace, health, power, good feelings and all powers, which exist in man, come out of his conscious. One, who lives in the sphere of consciousness, is calm even without money in his pocket. He is not afraid of anything, and concentrates his thinking on the sublime world. No more than an hour and a half, the help comes, bread comes, or the car comes. That man is wise and never abuses with his powers and abilities, which he has.

People think that no matter what food they eat, no matter how they think, they can be healthy. This is impossible. Health is connected to the clean thoughts and feelings, to the clean food of good quality.

The face of a saint shines. It is neither sallow and emaciated as you think, nor his eyes are deep-set.

One who is lean is not a saint, nor one who is stout.

When man thinks, the powers of the cerebrum go to the sympathetic nervous system, to the brain system. When these energies cross rightly, man is healthy, and thinks and feels normally.

Health is an internal process. If the organism is not healthy inside, no matter what favorable external conditions there are, he cannot use them. What is needed in order man to be healthy? First he shall determine his attitude to God, then to his soul and after that to his neighbor. If these relations are normal, man will be healthy.

The strength and health do not come from the external food. God feed man from inside and gives him power and life to work and solve his tasks. One, who eats a lot, pays a lot.

Health is a result from right exchange of the energies in man's organism, on one side, as well as of right exchange between the souls, on the other side. If a disease comes, it is a breach of the law of the right exchange.

In the healthy organism, the blood is distributed equally along all organs of the body and the energy, which comes out of the brain, has to be distributed also equally and the thoughts have to penetrate into all cells.

If the particles of the matter, of which the human organism is composed, are in normal relations between each other, all organs of his will be in harmony. When they are in harmony, man's feelings and deeds will be harmonious.

In order to maintain the harmony of his organism, man shall feed his brain with bright feelings, his heart – with clean feelings, his lungs – with clean air, his stomach – with clean wholesome food.

One, who wants to be healthy, shall increase the quantity of love and energy in him. Take more energy from the Sun, if you want to be cheerful. Enjoy the sunrise if you want to prolong your life.

The law of cleanness is one of the major laws of Life. The state of health of everybody and the cleanness of the soul depend on it. All diseases are results from dirtiness. Microbes exist in the physical world, as well as in the spiritual and mental worlds.

One, who wants to be healthy, not to be ailing, not to be irritable, shall be clean. Microbes do not affect one, who is clean. Therefore, if you want to be healthy, work on your body, get rid of all dirt and useless sediment and fats. If you notice that fat has accumulated somewhere along your body, apply a Spartan health regime right away.

Health is not possible without cleanness.

One in soul is such as he is in body and vice versa. Some people think that one may be ailing, and feeble, and yet - genial. This is impossible. One, who is genial, has a specific body structure. If he gets ill, he easily recovers.

Healthy person is the one, in whom each organ has its own tone and vibrations. As long as all man's organs function normally, pleasant and harmonious tones are produced by their activity. If the function of the human organs is correct and creates music, it may be said that one's health is in perfect state. Further, each musical tone has its own color.

What are the features, after which we can guess who is healthy? When man is healthy by body, heart and mind, three fragrances come out of him. The healthy body emanates a special pleasant fragrance. The sublime feelings emanate another type of fragrance. If one of the three fragrances is absent, one is ill in a certain aspect.

One is truly healthy, if he moves and is ready for work during the whole day. He does not know what a disease is. He does not complaints of anything. He is ready to help everybody.

How you can guess that one is healthy? When one, who is healthy, looks at the sky in the evening or during the day, he immediately feels happiness, joy, and thanks for everything that he has. One, who cannot rejoice when he looks at the sky and does not thank for all that it is given to him, is ill.

The healthy man has clean, clear, open sight, and established outlook. He vibrates of life, of the energy in him, enjoys the hardships in life.

Lots of people ask me why man shall be good. It is simple. Man shall be good in order to be healthy. Goodness, virtue is the first condition for man's health.

One, who has strong will is healthy. His blood is clean; his arms, legs, backbone are healthy. The healthy body is a result of strong, wise will.

First of all health depends on one's way of thinking. By knowing the laws of thinking and their right application, man can be healthy.

If you want to be healthy, you shall think of the healthy people. In general, man becomes what he thinks about.

Man is healthy when there are cold electrical flows on the right side, and on the left one – warm flows.

In order man to be healthy, his head shall be cool, and his feet warm. If the opposite happens, he has to find a way to change his state.

The more gold there is in the human blood, the more noble, stable and healthy he is.

Keep your nose in good state. Keep it and respect it as a sacred organ. While your nose in good state, man is healthy. As long as the nose is well, you shall know that the eyes, ears and mouth will be well. Therefore, lungs will be also well, as well as the heart and the stomach. If something spoils in the nose, the organism gradually disassembles. Keep your nose and do not be afraid. Watch for the curved line of the nostrils not to be smoothened. It is a misfortune if it smoothes out. It is a misfortune if you have no a nose. It is a nice mountain peak, where the energies of the human organism transform. One, who does not know the significance of the human nose, cannot evaluate it as a great blessing of life. While your nose is in good state, God will speak to you through your mind and your heart. Notice – the central place on the human face is taken by the nose. God manifests on the Earth in three ways: through man's thoughts, feelings and deeds. This imprints on the nose.

Your head shall be always upright. Never look downwards. The head and the backbone shall always be perpendicular to the earth. When you are upright you connect to the solar energies and positive things in life.

The head shall be always perpendicular to the Sun and the center of the Earth, In order the vibrations to be correctly perceived.

You shall know how to hold your head in relation to the center of the

Sun – you shall hold your head vertically in relation to the Sun and the Earth. In order you not to fall, dislocate a leg, break your head, you shall learn how to walk, stand and sit. If troubles frequently happen to you, it means that you do not know how to walk: your legs are not correctly positioned in relation to the center of the Earth, and your head is not correctly positioned in relation to the center of the Sun.

In the physical world, man shall keep the normal warmth of his organism. His health depends on it. In the spiritual he shall keep the internal fire, not to extinguish it. It is called "sacred fire".

In order the sacred fire to burn forever, it depends on the right circulation, right thoughts, feelings and deeds of man.

Reasons for Diseases

One, who does not know the reason of a disease, he cannot treat it. Each disease has its distant or close reason. By going along the right road of life, man easily solves his tasks, he does not breach the laws of Nature. Each breach or diversion leads to a disease. The diversion may have happened many years ago, but the consequences come today. One, who finds the reason of his disease, recovers easily. If he does not find it, the disease does not leave him.

Diseases are due to breaking of the Divine laws. One, who does not obey these laws, various sediments accumulate in his organism, in his stomach – various acids, and he gets ill.

Nature loves those, who follow its laws. It raises them, gives them life in abundance. One, who does not follow its laws – it considers him not fit to use its goods and deprives him from all civil rights of its kingdom. Such a man is exposed to lots of diseases and misfortunes.

You may treat yourselves, if you correct your sins. Your sins have created your diseases.

How is it explained that the reasons for diseases are spiritual? The negative or destructive thoughts or feelings initially are in the invisible bodies of man: astral, mental, etc. After that, they, with their vibrations, come down into the ether body, and from the ether body – into the physical one. When they come down to the physical body, they attack those organs, through their vibration, to which they are related in accordance with the character of their vibrations. They may attack the kidneys, the liver, the heart, and the lungs and destroy them or make them prone to diseases. And then, because of the smallest external reason, the organism gets ill.

Remember: each disease is a result from a committed crime in the past or presently. Not knowing that, doctors think that they can cope with the diseases. Till when will this continue? Till people come to the understanding to look for the reasons for the diseases in themselves and when they find them, to eliminate them.

There are two reasons for being ill: either you do not love, or you are not loved.

All diseases are due to sins and crimes. In order the doctor to be able to treat the ill person, he shall go deep in the reason of diseases. Nature sends diseases as a way of correcting the crimes.

Some people are scared of the law of inheritance, but this law is a blessing, because in this way, one sin, which is handed down to the fourth generation, is eliminated. One good thought is handed down to many generations, which means that the good is stronger than the evil. If you do not do another crime during that time, thousands of years you will benefit of one good deed. If you make a mistake and you do not correct it, your fortune will follow you from four to ten generations.

Sometimes when the father is a genius, the son is not. Fathers are weak in handing down their geniality to their children.

Mothers may hand down more things to their sons than their fathers.

Geniality is handed down by female line, by the line of feelings.

The reasons for diseases is hidden in the astral world, and the consequences manifest in the physical one. That is why people complaint of pains in the head, heart, lungs, stomach, etc. One, who wants to treat himself, first he shall find the reason for his illness in the astral world. When he eliminates the reason, the disease will leave him.

There are organic diseases, which hide their origin in man's distant past. When a disease embeds in the astral body, it gradually goes into the mind, and from there – to the physical body. In order man to recover, this disease shall go away from his mind. One bitter feeling or one inconsistent thought causes physical diseases. When the reason is removed, the disease disappears.

Many diseases are due to disorders in feelings. Many diseases are due to disorders in the mind. When the diseases are due to mental disorders, they affect the muscular system and the lungs. When the disorders are mainly of sensual character, they affect the heart, the liver, the respiratory system and the blood vessels.

Diseases and painful states are due to a lack of music and harmony in man.

If you have a headache, the reason is in the stomach. If you have a stomachache, the reason is in the head. Diseases come after the law of reflection.

There is one internal thread in Nature, which passes the good and evil features of the whole Life. This law exists in each man, too. If you have a look at somebody, you will see that he is entangled in threads of the darkness and of the light. When one of the dark threads passes round him, he will be in bad state. If one of the light threads comes by him, he will be in good state.

The mixing of the dark threads with the light ones constantly creates the good and bad states. The threads of the light shall surmount the ones of the darkness. The nice, bright, noble, and moral feelings are creations of the threads of the light.

There are invisible creatures, in the interest of which is they to excite the energies in man, in order to benefit from him. When one is angry, they use that energy and make him powerless. I watch how these creatures come. They come in groups, sit round the man and begin to impose on him negative thoughts till they predispose him. When they achieve their aim, they go away and watch what he will do.

Behind each disease, creatures of different level of development are hidden: strong or weak, good or bad. Most of them are bad, with low culture. This is not a scientific explanation for diseases, but a delusion for many people. In spite of this, I say: behind each disease, creatures, which have dropped behind in their spiritual development, are hidden.

When the parents quarrel, children become ailing. Where there is love between the parents, children are healthy.

If you make a mistake, you will feel a pain either in the stomach, in the heart, in the lungs, or in the legs, or in the elbow, or in the intestines, or in the toes, or in the backbone, or in the liver – the localization of the diseases in the various places show what kind of a mistake you have made. Nature has a particular medicine.

If you have laughed at somebody's illness, that illness will surely visit you. Find the person at whom you have laughed and apologize him. When you apologize and prove that you understand the situation of the ones, who suffer, the illness will leave you.

When somebody hates you, he sends, through his eyes, fiery waves towards you and if your nervous system is upset, something bad may reach you. Some people curse and their words are so strong that their curses may happen and the said words may hit.

Many of your states and diseases are somebody else's, adopted by you through suggestion. You have seen somebody with a broken leg, you have experienced his state and after a while the same place is painful for you. As the pain has come after a suggestion, it has to go away in the same way.

The Earth, as a living creature, has its own horoscope, its own path, along which it walks. Its path now is not as smooth as it used to be earlier. Sometimes the Earth passes through certain perturbations. People often are infected with these influences of the Earth and the various epidemic diseases occur in this way. Thousands and millions of people die from these diseases.

A doctor comes, hurries through the patient, feels his pulse, writes down a recipe and goes out. One is not treated in this way. There are diseases, which result from discouragement, overwork, cold. The reason may be the back part of the brain. Some diseases may result from the destructive abilities, others – from too much or random eating. Some diseases may be also a result from mixing of heterogeneous food, others – from a split between the mind and heart; third ones – from breaking of the law of love and thousands of reasons more may be listed. If the law of faith is broken, the nervous system upsets. If there is a split between the sympathetic nervous system and the brain nervous system, disorder is again caused. If one gets discouraged, if he loses hope, disagreement appears between the muscles and the bones. More blood comes to some places, and more energy gathers at others. Some diseases are due to the reason that man has come into clash with people or into clash with himself. So, it is not easy at all to be a real doctor, and not only a doctor with a label or a company.

The reason for the rheumatism is not the moisture in the room. If the moisture was the reason for the rheumatism, how you are going to explain the illness of somebody, who lives in a hygienic, comfortable environment, where there is no moisture? All diseases in the world are results from the breach of God's law.

The reason of each disease shall be looked for far away. If we live after a Divine way, a day will come, when our bodies will be right away cleaned of all kinds of dregs, which cause diseases today. Some physicists consider that if electricity of 10 - 20 thousand of volts or 100 000 volts is applied to the human organism, it would renovate in a very short time.

If you retain a Divine desire in yourself, you consciously block yourself, as a result of which you expose yourselves to lots of diseases. All diseases are results of exactly that blocking, caused by non-fulfillment of the Divine desires, which make you do good.

People get ill only because they break their connection with the Divine world, as a result of which they deprive themselves of the energies of that world.

There is satiety in the material world, in the spiritual one and in the Divine one. The world is full of surfeited people. All diseases originate from the satiety.

While one obeys God's laws, each cell in his organism is subject to renovation. When he stops obeying these laws, his cells begin to destroy gradually. Each negative thought, each negative feeling causes specific shocks, specific explosions in the cells of the human organism. These shocks affect painfully his organism. The reason for all diseases is hidden in the human wicked and negative thought.

Human thoughts penetrate in the intermolecular space of the brain nervous system, and the feelings – into the interatomic space of the sympathetic nervous system. This is exactly the difference between the human thoughts and feelings. If one blocks a thought of his, i.e. if he does not allow it to implement, it will cause an explosion in the brain nervous system. And if he blocks a feeling of his, it will cause an explosion in the sympathetic nervous system.

Many people complain of the intense sun and say that it affects their organs badly. The reason for that is not the Sun, but their thoughts and feelings. Bad thoughts and feelings form a dark zone round the Sun, which refracts the solar beams so that it retains a big part of them – the so called black light of the Sun. These black beams are the reason for lots of diseases, as well as for the blackening of the people. It may be concluded from here that the origin of all diseases is hidden in a specific internal refraction of the solar light. Light, which refracts in a descending order, always produces painful states in the human organism.

Never stay in the shadow of a tree or in the shadow of somebody else. This is a rule, which may be tried by everybody. Many diseases are due to shadows. Each beam, which has reached a man, is evaporated by his organism and after that it comes out again in the form of a dead light. In the shadow of the flower, of the tree or in the shadow of the house, there is still light under the effect of the direct solar beams, and not of the indirect, i.e. the beams of the shadow. Never stay in shadow. Nothing grows in it.

Man cannot keep a certain idea in his mind without it to produce a certain physiological effect on his brain and his nervous system. Knowing the power of the thoughts, of the feelings and of your deeds, you shall be careful about them. One thought, one feeling, one word may cause in the brain and heart of somebody such a tension that it can cripple him.

There is no a stronger poison than the negative thoughts, feelings and states of somebody. Fear, hatred, doubt, suspicion are such poisons. They are dregs, which accumulate in blood and poison it. May man be healthy at such states?

Disharmonious thoughts upset the brain nervous system; disharmonious feelings upset the sympathetic nervous system, and the disharmonious deeds upset the muscle and bone systems. The physical and psychic lives are closely connected.

Our unclean thoughts and desires sometimes leave dregs in our consciousness, as a result of which lots of painful states occur. These dregs accumulate on the spiritual body of man and produce internal perturbations.

Some diseases are nothing else, but a result from spells from the past. For each mischief, wickedness or injustice, done to somebody, man perceives his dissatisfaction and spell, which introduces disharmony in his organism and predisposition to diseases. The wishes of people to their fellows, not matter good or bad, reach them finally. Human thoughts are powerful.

The way the cart shakes somebody, in the same way the vibrations of rude words, of negative thoughts and feelings cause shaking to the nervous system.

It is awful for somebody to keep bad thoughts about somebody else in his mind. Mendacious thoughts accumulate on the consciousness of man as dregs and cause him lots of troubles and sufferings. Negative thoughts make man nervous and indisposed. In order to get rid of bad and negative thoughts, one shall work on his self-education.

While thinking, man knows the place of each word and never smears his language. As long as his language is clean, his body will be healthy. If he introduces one unclean word in his language, he smears his thinking. As long as his thinking is smeared, he introduces poison in his organism and after a while he gets ill.

Each bad word affects badly the liver. Hygiene forbids man to use negative and disharmonious words. As long as one goes against the hygiene, he upsets his liver. As long as the liver is upset, the nervous system upsets, too, as well as the digestion. In general, bad words affect health badly. If you want to be healthy, use good, positive words.

Warmth and light, which are formed by the human feelings and thoughts, affect the organism either favorably or destructively. This depends on their vibrations. The higher and more their vibrations are, the more favorable their effect on the human organism is.

Each unpleasant thought is nothing else, but a wandering soul, which has made a sin on the Earth, was not able to finish its development and now it cannot find a place for itself. Sing a song, have a talk. All sad thoughts, which attack you, are suffering souls, which stay tied between the physical and astral worlds and cannot develop.

Man shall think only 50% for himself (this shall be the maximum) and 50% about his fellows, if he wants to fulfill God's law. One shall not be negligent of himself, but he cannot neglect his fellows either. As a result of this diseases occur.

When one's brain activity increases, the activity of the physical body decreases. This is the reason for the big number of nervous people at the present. The larger the brain activity is, the weaker man is. In order his nervous system not to get exhausted, part of his mental powers shall be poured into the heart. The powers of the organism are a result from the sum of the powers of the mind and of the heart.

If you look for the reason of the illness of the ears and of the eyes, you will find it in the back part of the brain. When the functions of the back part of the brain does not happen in the right way, man suffers of pain in the ears and in the eyes. When the temporal part of the brain does not function correctly, man complains of pains in the mouth. Knowing that the brain is the reason for lots of diseases, keep it in good shape. When we are talking of good shape of the brain, we have in mind the thoughts, which pass through it. That is why we shall hold the thoughts responsible for the state of health of the brain, and for the state of health of the heart – the feelings. Each thought brings either good or poison to man. The same concerns man's feelings and desires. In addition, there are thoughts, which show their effect on the organism right away, and others – after a while.

I say: introduce into the mind of even the strongest man two controversial thoughts and he will by no means go out of his mind. They cause enormous shaking of the nervous system, disturbance of the internal harmony, or, said in an occult language, going of the human doppelganger out of the body. Another creature takes its place. One, who understands the laws, may turn back the doppelganger and restore the normal state of the man.

Two reasons may cause weakening of the eyes: worries and incorrect thoughts. If they can be overcome, the eyesight will improve. God has not created man with glasses.

The reason for weakening of the eyesight is that today's people have no deep philosophical thinking like the first people – the people of the ancient wisdom. Today people live without knowing why they live. They are embarrassed. They do not know what the day of tomorrow will bring them. What are you going to answer to the question: "Why do you live?" We live in order to improve ourselves. We live for God. If they put you to an exam, will you pass it? When one lives for an idea, he is ready for all sacrifices. That is why the idea, because of which one is ready for all sacrifices, shall deserve that.

Man's eyes serve his mind. While his mind functions normally, his eyes will be in good shape. If his mind begins to weaken, one's physical strength begins gradually to weaken. Man, in whom charity works, has always healthy eyes and ears.

Why does one become blind? It is because he has not lived in accordance with the laws of the rational nature. When one worries too much, the anxiety produces concussion first to his stomach system. The concussion is transferred to the lungs from there, from the lungs – to the brain, and from the brain – to the optic nerve. When the optic nerve weakens, man begins gradually to lose his eyesight. In order to restore his eyesight, one shall start to restore the normal state of his organs in a reverse order: first of the brain, then – of the lungs and finally – of the stomach, from where the concussion has originated. After that he has to find the reason for the concussion and eliminate it.

According to the occultism, all blind people, all disabled people, whom we meet today on the Earth, are all students, who have not passed their examinations, as a result of which they have left the school.

That neurasthenia, which exists all over Europe, is a loosening of the white race. All minds are full only of thoughts about houses, money, conveniences. Material goods have replaced the clean thoughts and clean desires, which give powers to man.

If one, who is pious, worries, he will lose his health. If a sinner does not worry and keeps his internal peace, he will always be healthy. God has given brain to man to think and not to worry.

It is noticed that good thoughts and feelings have a favorable effect on the digestive system, and bad ones – unfavorable. Voracity and the enormous man's desire for pleasure upset his stomach system. When the stomach does not work, one's brain system upsets, too. If you meet somebody with a dry face, yellow and indisposed to work, you shall know that his stomach system is not in good shape. He cannot work. He takes a gloomy view of everything. He has no faith in life.

Headache is due to breaking of the laws of the right thought. Correct your thinking and the headache will disappear.

Irritability and nervousness are due to an excessive brain energy, which accumulates in the nose. The excessive brain energy upsets the nervous system, hence, do not overwork your mind by useless worries and little things.

You ask: what is the reason for the misfortunes in our lives? One of the important reasons for that is the promiscuous killing of mammals, of people. When the souls of the killed go to the astral world, they introduce conditions for nerve diseases and disorders amongst people. The killed criminal moves freely amongst weak-willed people and suggest them feelings for revenge.

Certain diseases, bad thoughts and desires, which manifest in you, are causes by some mammals. In order you to get rid of these sufferings, you shall mild your attitude towards the animals. Often the hatred of a dog may have the same effect as the hatred of a man. Do not think that the thoughts of the animals are too weak. No, they are very dangerous for the world.

Good man has healthy legs; impartial man has healthy arms; wise man has healthy ears; and one, who loves the truth, has healthy eyes. If one loves God, his mind will be also well developed.

When one loses and abandons one of his virtues, he simultaneously loses that organ, which serves this virtue. And when he sinks in the sphere of the sin, man gradually begins to atrophy: the legs, the arms and the rest organs.

Today people suffer of various diseases and by not knowing the reason for their manifestation, they cannot heal themselves. The reasons for the diseases are psychic. For example, the reason for a tumor hides in the perversion of the manifestations of love. If avidity occurs in someone, this shows that a certain number of cells in the organism differentiate, want to live separately, to disobey the common order in the organism. In this way, they create their own lodging and form a new country with free government. They work in this way for days, months, years, while the doctor does not come with his artillery against these disobedient citizens and begins to bomb them. Sometimes he succeeds in making them go outside, and sometimes complications occur, which direct man to the other world. However, there is another way for treatment – through grafting. In the way it is done with fruit trees, grafting may be also done in man's organism, in order saps to be made go upwards. When the energies in the living organism stop, at the place, where this happens, a certain bump appears, which doctors call a tumor. Hence, one, who understands the laws of grafting, he will be able in one or another way to direct the energies in the organism to flow through the bump, too. When they begin to flow through it, it disappears completely. If the new cells manage to take the saps of the cells, which form the tumor, it will not have conditions for development and it will completely disappear.

If you all serve love, there will not be ill people. If you have rheumatism, you love is not enough. Each disease is due to an internal insufficiency or to lack of light, or to lack of goodness, or to lack of power.

Human love shall be always cleaned. Otherwise it introduces dirt in the organism. It is a reason for the unclean blood in the organism. To purify human love means to replace it by the Divine one.

You cannot love and be ill. These are two incompatible things. As long as you love, your face cannot be dark, your eyes cannot be blurred. Love bears life.

Phosphorous decreases in the brain, because love has decreased. All elements, which exist at the physical field, are submitted to love, as well as to those elements, of which the spiritual and mental worlds are formed.

When hope in man decreases, diseases come. When faith decreases – other diseases come. When Love decreases, the worst diseases come. When you increase them, the diseases will go away.

People get ill, because they have broken the law of truth. One, who wants to correct his life and restore his health, he has to come to love the truth.

Pride is the reason for many diseases. All diseases are healed through humility. Man gets free of painful states through humility.

Each physical defect is due to spiritual reasons. If you hate someone, your chests will suffer, a disease will occur there. If you feel envious, your heart will suffer. From envy, jealousy, doubt, suspicion, the liver will suffer. If you indulge yourselves too much in eating, your stomach will get ill. If you get angry, constipation will begin. If you promise and do not fulfill, headache comes. When you find the reason for the illness, balance will be restored, harmony will be established.

When you have a headache, you shall strive to correct your attitude to the Divine world. If you have a chestache, you shall correct your attitude to the spiritual world. If you have a stomachache, you shall correct your attitude to the physical world. Each man's disease has its deep reasons, it is not random. Contemporary science and medicine do not look for the internal reasons of things. They consider all phenomena in Nature and life in their internal material side. What is the reason for the stitches at certain parts of the body? They are due to shrinking of the capillaries. It is known that the capillaries serve for the circulation. They bring love to all parts of the body. When the capillaries in the zone of the chest shrink, the electricity in the organism, which bears light, cannot function properly along the entire organism, as a result of which in certain zones more of it accumulates, like the water vapor in a steam-boiler, and causes stitches. Often the atmospheric electricity connects to the electricity of the human organism and a small explosion happens, which is felt as pain by man. What shall you do in order you to get rid of the stitches? Introduce more warmth in your organism. This means to change the state of your feelings and in this way you send more blood to that part of your bodies, in which you feel stitches. When that part gets warm, the stitches go away. Hence, man can cure himself by a strong mind, by strong and positive feelings, as well as by hot water.

Man shall live normally; obey the laws of nature, in order capillaries not to shrink too much. Shrinking causes infection, and from there – various bumps, stitches, fainting-fits, etc. Each bad thought, each bad feeling and bad deed shrinks the capillaries and stops the flows of electricity and magnetism in human organism. Their rhythms change. Disharmony establishes and man gets ill.

People are a system of interconnected vessels, according to which if one gets ill or suffers, thousands of people get ill or suffer together with him.

Nature uses symbols and imprints. There is no a crime or good, which is done by somebody and which is not imprinted by nature on his body. It marks all crimes and all virtues.

Each disease is due to a spiritual reason. The incorrect relations between close people – a mother and children, brothers and sisters, a man and a woman – cause various diseases. When they correct their relations, the disease disappears.

If there is disagreement between a man and a woman in one home, children will by no means be often ill. Children are healthy and well educated, when the mother and the father live in harmony.

Some women do not have children, because they did not have to marry or have married too early.

If a son comes into a clash with his father and his father's mind is stronger than his, the son will go away quicker than the father. If you hate your mother, she will go away sooner. If your mother hates you, you will not live long. You shall love your mother, father, brother, and sister from a healthy point of view, because if you provoke them through your hatred, their thoughts toward you will destroy you. It is possible, when you hate and when you are hated, to fence yourselves constantly by prayers and formulas.

In that case, it is better to use the law of Love and when it is recommended to love your fellow, it is for people to be healthy. If everybody loves each other in a family, diseases do not come in such a home. And if they come, they go away quickly.

If we break our connections with the animals, our stomach system will upset right away, and as a result of this our state of health will change. Do not get rid of the animal in yourselves – the animals maintain the stomach system. You shall be sensible and create right relations with the animals. There are three worlds (animal, human and angelic), which are in a certain internal ratio, in a certain dependence. Hence, the stomach shall be in harmony with the lungs, and the lungs – with the brain. The sense is not in getting rid of the animal, but to regulate it, educate it, submit the lower desires and feelings to the higher ones.

The reason for all ulcers in the stomach is always the lie. The lie changes the chemical composition of the blood and of the tissues of the organism. How is this change in the organism explained? By fear. When one lies, he begins to fear and this lie causes shrinking of the blood vessels, as well as of the tissues.

Each surfeit in the physical, spiritual or mental world leads to satiation. Satiation is the reason for lots of painful states. It is said that man shall work more, but not too much. It is not allowed satiation in work, too. Man shall work until it is pleasant to him. Real work is the one, which organizes one's powers.

There is a state, which you do not realize, and it is the fact that you only take. You want only good, and you give nothing. In that case, evil is as a process of depriving you of what you take.

You shall give, in order to clean yourself.

You shall give, in order to rejuvenate.

You shall give, in order to grow. You shall give, in order to be healthy.

One, who loves, gives. God always gives.

The Divine law means constant giving.

Why do people become mad? When people are close, a clash happens between them. When they clash, their doppelgangers may entangle, because of which one of them may lose his mind.

All, who lead vicious lives, get mad. Getting mad is allowable for a disturbed nervous system, for a vicious way of life. You shall know this. But, for a man, who has leaded a clean life, getting mad is absolutely impossible.

The reason for getting mad of contemporary people is hidden in their past existences. Today they come upon a case for getting mad, but the actual reason is hidden in them.

Sufferings, which contemporary people experience, are due to their gluttony. Sufferings show that each man has taken more of the goods than he needs.

The neck shall not be full, because there are glands in it, which fulfill various functions and it shall not be fat, in order these glands to execute the work properly.

If too many fats accumulate there, various chest diseases occur, the tonsils get ill and lots of other diseases, connected with the improper functioning of these glands, appear.

Cancer, tumors, of which people suffer today, are due to opposition or controversial feelings, to disharmony between the cerebrum and the sympathetic nervous system, to vicious life, to greediness. A disease locates where gluttony is. It is needed deep internal unity, harmony, bathes with solar water, bathing in the violet color, onion to be eaten every day, as well as new tissue, new cells to be grafted in the same way, in which grafting is done with a tree.

Men, women, children – they are all nervous. Why? Because of their crimes. "My mother has born me a neurasthenic" – some people say. No, you, with your vicious life, has created your neurasthenia.

When does one become nervous? When he bears a larger load than his capabilities.

What is the reason of neurasthenia? The outgoing of the doppelganger. The doppelganger often goes out 1-2 cm, and sometimes more. When it goes out more than it is necessary, one becomes extremely impatient. In order not to lose his temper, he shall armor himself. Mildness is armor for man. That is why I say: the more sensitive man becomes, the more milder language he shall have.

Contemporary people have become neurasthenics, because they are often angry. I say: if you want to heal your neurasthenia, stop getting angry. How? You will apply your will.

The upset of the liver causes lots of diseases. For example, neurasthenia is also due to an upset of the liver. Correct your liver, in order to correct your mind. The upset of the liver affects the mental abilities and man's feelings, as well as his spiritual manifestations. Under liver I understand the activity of the lower worlds in man. The lower feelings influence the liver like the termites, which eat everything.

Neurasthenia is due to cracks in the nervous system, from where the nervous energy flows outside. Fear also causes cracks in the nervous system. In order to get rid of neurasthenia, one shall stop the flowing-outs of the nervous energy.

Many people get ill of neurasthenia due to the warmth, which certain types of feelings produce in the back part of the brain. This warmth affects badly the stomach system, as well as the lungs. The treatment of those people happens through turning of the thermal energy into magnetism, which raises the vital power of the organism. There are doctors – magnetizers, who liberate man from the harmful for the organism warmth. Water, taken in homeopathic dose, plays a major role in that treatment. If it enters in this way in the brain, it reduces the burning and one, who is ill, recovers. In order a treatment to be effective, the doctor shall have a diploma from the living nature, except the one from the medical faculty. And namely the powers of his organism shall be in harmony with the powers of the rational nature.

If the feelings and desires of somebody are not satisfied, he becomes a neurasthenic. Put an obstacle in front of the realization of somebody's strives and desires and you will see that soon he will become a neurasthenic. Remove the obstacle from his path, and neurasthenia will disappear.

The larger the desires are, the bigger the sufferings are.

When man's desires are not regulated, anger comes: anger is energy, which is not used properly.

Man is free until he accepts a desire in himself and it submits him. When he accepts it and begins to feed it, he loses his freedom. Each desire out of you is a manifestation of a creature, which stands lower or higher than you and influences you. If you connect to that desire, you connect to the creature, from which it comes and you cannot get rid of it for a long time. Each desire in man is a connection with other creatures, which live outside of him and that connection is not only external. It hides it roots deep in the human nature.

Contemporary people complain of indisposition of the spirit, of exhaust, of nervousness. Which is the reason for these states? The reason is their numerous desires. They have many desires, and little soil. In order to grow up and give fruits, plant needs earth.

If one does not know how to transform properly the energies of his lower desires, he may get ill. This disease will affect his feelings and his spiritual life. That is why, together with the anatomy and physiology of the physical body, one shall study the anatomy and physiology of the astral body. Diseases of contemporary people are due to not understanding of the law of transforming of the energies.

You walk and wave with your arms, talk and wave with your arms. You shall cope with the unnatural movements. You knit your brows, purse your lips, narrow your eyes – with this unnatural movements you misrepresent your features. You worry and you frown and you cause harm to yourselves.

When people are very nervous, more glucose remains in the blood. Joyful, well disposed people do not have glucose in the blood. The numerous desires also increase the blood glucose.

Hairs have grown up under the influence of warmth. When warmth begins to decrease, hairs fall away and the head becomes bald. Hair fall is due to lack of warmth, which is connected with magnetism. Hair falls as a result of loss of magnetism, of many worries, of painful states, of heavy diseases.

When the head begins to become bald, the mind gains mastery also over the heart, the brain is extremely active.

Ungratefulness cripples and makes one look older prematurely, and gratefulness revives, raises and rejuvenates. Why do people get ill? Because they are ungrateful. What shall we do in order to recover? Apply gratefulness to your life. Be grateful for the smallest good, which is given to you.

Sometimes, at a sin, 50-60 thousand cells may die, and other times – even up to 100 thousand cells. At a big worry, at big desperation, thousands of cells die in the organism.

All mental diseases originate from the insufficiency of light. All heart diseases originate from the insufficiency of warmth. All diseases of the soul originate from the insufficiency of truth.

Doubt is the one of the most dangerous parasites, which propagates quickly. Within 24 hours it is capable of poisoning man's blood and after that he shall make big efforts in order to clean his blood again.

Treatment shall start 20 years before the disease has appeared. Future doctors will treat ill people even before they have got ill. What kind of a disease is cancer and what is the reason for it? The reasons for the cancer are in the contrast of feelings. When somebody begins to lead a vicious life, he will by no means get ill of cancer. When man gives up the higher idea, which has inspired him in his life, he will by no means get a chest disease and he will become a pessimist. Tuberculosis appears in this way.

The more unrestrained the feelings of somebody are, the weaker his memory is. Human memory weakens also because of big sufferings, of big fear and of strong mental shocks.

One, who suffers of palpitation, is a haughty man. One, who suffers of stomachache, is also haughty. One, who suffers of headache, is vain.

The reasons for the palpitation are psychic. These reasons have formed lots of poisons, which have entered the organism. They are alien elements, semiorganic substances, which have to go out of the organism. Palpitation is due to controversial thoughts, feelings and desires, which are useless for the heart. There are various methods for getting rid of them. One of the new ways for healing is music. There are pains, which can be healed by playing a violin, others – a guitar, a flute, etc. The various instruments has different effect on each separate man. You shall treat the heart by songs, which begin with the tone "C", taken not by pitchfork, but the natural one. If the major tone "C" is taken correctly, man may obtain vital energy from the Sun and transfer it to all organs. When one, who is ill sings, he establishes conditions in himself for treatment.

If you feel palpitation, this shows that there is bifurcation in your feelings. Palpitation is a result of a struggle between two feelings. Eliminate the struggle and palpitation will disappear.

There is a danger of satiety while eating. In the same way, there is a danger of stupefying of feelings at big joy. The way human nervous system is created, it is not capable of withstanding the vibrations of the big higher joy, experienced by the higher creatures. If one comes upon the vibrations of such a joy, the nervous system, as well as his brain, will upset, because it is not fit for withstanding neither the higher, nor the lower vibrations of some creatures.

With the efforts of the will, you will strengthen also your body. All organs will start to work well. The weakening of the will is a condition for a disease. Diseases are needed for strengthening of the will.

If one organ develops at the expense of another one, if some cells rejuvenate at the expense of others, various diseases like cancer, tumor, etc. appear. When some abilities and feelings develop at the expense of others, the organism gets ill, too.

The legs become cold with some people. Introduce love into yourself. You will have warmth even at the end of your toes. If your toes become cold, then your love has bankrupted.

Incorrect feelings affect the circulation. If your feelings improve, it will also improve and thanks to that the arms and legs will also become warmer.

The thing, which Bulgarians call "uroki" (a spell), is due to the fact that man has stepped on a blade of grass or a plant, by which he has caused harm to it.

Nowadays people are afraid of all epidemic diseases, and are not afraid of the sins and crimes, which are the reasons for these diseases.

The first reason for the anomalies in life is the unnatural food, which you put in your stomachs. God has made man to eat fruits, and you eat meat. The meat diet has introduced such poisons in your organism, that it is an assembly of impurities today. If you had uncorrupted sense of smell, you should run away from each other – such a stink comes out of those, who eat meat. If somebody is ailing, the first condition for him to get better is to improve his food. Fruits and meat contain different elements, which evoke two different states, which will produce two different results in the far future of our lives.

Contemporary people suffer when they eat meat. Only one microscopic part of the food is assimilated, and the other part is an excess. This excess shall be thrown outside. All diseases nowadays are due to that excess, and in spite of that everybody preach that more food is needed. No, man needs less food and it shall be accepted and assimilated so that the least possible excess to remain from it.

When food is not digested well, blood is not being well purified either. Then semiorganic matter accumulates round the joints in the form of sediments. These improper things in the organism create indisposition of the spirit, pessimism. In order not to fall into pessimism, through the power of your will, work for the improvement of your stomach system.

If today people are ill, nervous, suffering, this is partly because of the food they eat. They get benefit of the fruits of the earth, which is saturated with the blood of thousands and millions of victims – people and animals. The earth is saturated with human blood and it shall be cleaned. It may be cleaned only when it passes through the Divine fire – the fire of love.

Neurasthenia of today's people is due to the enormous consumption of meat. The only healthy food for today's people is the vegetarian one. It makes milder his rough nature. In future mankind will reach such a degree of development that they will be able to obtain the needed nourishing substances directly from the living nature and that food will be clean, perfect and completely healthy. At that phase of development, there will be no animals on the Earth.

When one eats unnatural food, lots of sediments gather in him. They attract the bacilli of various diseases – cholera, plague, classical typhus and others. Not all people, however, die of those diseases, because their blood is clean. One, who is clean, never gets ill. One, who is clean and has faith, may walk amongst choleric people and gets ill of nothing.

If one suffers from ill stomach, no matter how little food he takes, part of it can be never digested and is accumulated in the form of semiorganic substances round the joints and round the vertebrae of the backbone and causes complications in the organism. According to medicine, these are "rheumatic diseases", and in a spiritual language – "spiritual thorns".

When food is not well digested, it does not penetrate in blood and it cannot feed cells. It accumulates in the form of sediments round the joints, as well as in the capillaries - this is the reason for one, who gets ill of rheumatic fever. The longer food stays in the mouth, the easier part of the nourishing substances and of the food are absorbed. In this way they go directly in the nervous system. Those juices, which are not absorbed in the mouth, go directly to the stomach, where complete digestion takes place.

What is the reason for the headache? The reason is eating of hardly digestible food, which leaves excesses in the stomach. Then the stomach is not cleaned properly, as a result of which headache appears, and the stomach and the mouth begin to stink.

The reason for the headache hides in the small and large intestines. When they are not in good shape, man suffers of headache. In order to cope with the headache, first he shall put his legs in hot water, and after that clean his intestines. When he unburdens his intestines and stomach, the headache stops.

Dizziness hides its reasons in the stomach.

Sometimes you feel heaviness in your stomach, but you do not know the reason for that. If you are acquainted with the functions of the sympathetic nervous system, you will understand that this heaviness, that indisposition in the stomach zone is related to your feelings, to your sympathetic nervous system. You have eaten some food, the vibrations of which does not correspond to the ones of your sympathetic nervous system, as a result of which certain disharmony appears. When this painful state goes away in a way, you begin to feel mental indisposition. Hence, the pain has transferred to the head, in the temporal zone, where you feel big tension. That is why one shall be careful about what he eats and what food is needed for his organism.

Surfeit is a blockage of the nervous system, and from there circulation becomes improper and the brain energy does not flow out and come in properly. Then a process of hardening of the joints occurs, at which they lose their plasticity. Finally the human spirit is forced to leave the body.

Bulgarians suffer of surfeit. If they eat less, everything will get better. When one eats, he shall reach to 20 bites and stop there.

Diseases are caused by the inert matter in man, but behind that matter a rational creature is hidden – good or bad. Some diseases destroy the human organism, and others purify it. You will say that you do not see the rational creature that hides behind the inert matter. This is another matter. You see that somebody is stabbed by knife and falls down. The knife is the inert matter, but the hand of a rational creature, which directs the knife, hides behind it. Rational creatures also hide behind the microbes, which cause various diseases and which affect the man in such a way that they create conditions, at which bacteria develop. In order to be able to guess which food is clean and healthy, watch for its effect on your thoughts, feelings and deeds. If the food introduces a certain decrease of the mental life of somebody, it is not hygienic. For example, people like pork meat, they eat it with pleasure, but it introduces such thoughts and moods, of which it is hard to get rid. Food affects mainly weak people with unorganized powers. It cannot influence much rational people. They know what food to eat.

In order to restore your memory, you shall liberate the brain of the accumulated in it lactic acid. How to get rid of it? By cleaning of the brain, of the blood in the whole organism. It is achieved by change of the food, by clean thoughts, by clean feelings and deeds.

The reason for the diseases hides in the blocked pores. The diseases occur in the zone of the organism, where blockage occurs. The organism does not bear any unclean things, any alien substances. If such unclean things gather somewhere, the organism gets ill. Each disease aims at liberating the organism from the alien substances. If any of the small channels in the backbone is blocked, one loses his vitality. The backbone has the property of absorbing the prana (or the vital energy) from the air and transfer it to the entire organism.

When the circulation of somebody is not normal, the carbon accumulates in the organism in the form of carbon dioxide and makes it unclean. When the electrical and magnetic energy does not flow properly in the human organism, then an excess of nitrogen accumulates in the nervous system, as a result of which the organism is blocked, which impedes the functions of the respiratory system.

If the eyes become yellow, the liver does not function well. The liver is related to the digestion. Digestion – to circulation, and blood cleanness depends on the latter. Unclean blood blurs the mind, distorts thinking.

The coldness of the legs is due to unclean blood in the organism. Unclean blood produces electricity in the organism, and the clean one - magnetism. Electricity produces cold, and magnetism - warmth.

The more unclean one's blood is, the worse he is.

By purifying your blood by deep breathing, you will find a way for purifying of your thoughts. Diseases are due to unclean blood and unclean food, which introduces unclean things in the stomach, which gradually poison the blood. The unclean blood bears diseases, causes indisposition, pessimism, laziness. One, who has clean blood, distinguishes with much energy and liveliness.

One, who breaths through the mouth, cannot be healthy.

By studying the processes of the human organism, you notice that some of the energies go out of the center of each cell and go outside in the space. Other energies come from outside and direct to the center of the cell. The place, where these energies meet, the activity in life is performed. If one of these flows of energies (the external or the internal) is blocked, various painful states occur in the organism. Each blockage destroys the normal circulation. As long as the circulation is not normal, the organism is exposed to various diseases.

The accumulation of solar energy in some parts of the body in larger quantity creates lots of painful states for the rest organs. In general, the organs, that get ill, are deprived of the needed quantity of energy. In order they to be healed, the needed energy has to be transferred to them mentally.

You have to study the laws of transforming the energy of one organ into another. All diseases of the organism are due to the not equal distribution of the energies in it, as a result of which the circulation is not normal.

Why do we suffer of headache? The headache is due to accumulation of cosmic energies in the brain.

The form of today's people is nothing but prana in movement. When the prana is not equally distributed in the human body, diseases occur, and when the prana is not equally distributed in feelings, dissatisfaction occurs, when prana is not equally distributed in thoughts, senselessness is born.

Physical roughening begins with roughening of the skin, which is a conductor of the vital energies in nature. When the skin roughens, the flow of these energies becomes improper and one gets ill. Skin roughening does not mean tanning, cracking or hardening. The symptoms are other.

If we are able to look with the eyes of a clairvoyant at the nerves and arteries of a neurasthenic, we will see cracks at lots of places, out of which the energy flows away. Such a man is weak. What are the reasons for that? First of all, these are the unbridled human passions.

The reason for getting insane is due to the fact that both parts of the brain are positive or negative. In order one to be in normal state, positive energy shall flow in one of the brain hemispheres, and in the other - negative. When one becomes too sharp, i.e. too electrical, mildness shall be applied to the left part of his brain, i.e. magnetism. If you put your hand on the head of a healthy man, you will feel two flows: one warm and one cold. However, if you put your hand on the head of an unstable man, you will feel only one warm flow. In order to help himself, he shall ask a friend of his, to put his hand on his head in order to regulate the energies of his brain.

Aim at transforming the excessive energy in yourselves, especially the one in the back part of the brain. That energy is the reason for almost all diseases, for all negative states. Sometimes that energy gathers behind the ears, as well as round the temporal zone and make one nervous, irritable, ready to be cross and take offence at the smallest thing.

One of the reasons for neurasthenia is the weak connection between the human organism and the solar energies. If you strengthen that connection, the neurasthenia will disappear. One, who is connected to the Sun, leads a good, rational, and moral life.

Through self-control, one assimilates the excessive energy of his organism. The neurasthenic, however, cannot assimilate that excessive energy in himself, as a result of which it disperses, flows out. Neurasthenia is due to cracks in the nervous system, from where the nervous energy flows out. Fear also evokes cracks in the nervous system, which causes outflow of nervous energy. In order to get rid of neurasthenia, one shall stop the outflow of nervous energy.

Which is the reason for the diseases? The reason is the weakening of the vital energy of somebody, at which it turns into potential and passive. In order to cure himself, one shall turn the potential energy into kinetic one. This can be achieved through various medications, which stimulate the passive energy. Sometimes Bulgarians treat the fever by splashing the ill person with cold water. In this way they produce a strong reaction and if the passive energy turns into active one, the ill person recovers.

Cough is a cold, and the cold shows that the organism has lost its initial vital power or the vibrations, at which the health may manifest. Raise your thought toward God, contact Him and the cough will disappear. There is only one Doctor in the world. All the rest are only His assistants.

Cough always comes from demagnetization of the organism. Demagnetization may be partial or total. If one organ gets ill, it gets demagnetized. The throat, lungs or the entire body may be demagnetized. Then we feel one big weakness and the magnetism of the organism shall be restored.

If you catch a cold, look for the reason of the disease. You will see that the reason is hidden in the superiority of the negative energies in the organism. And then it remains nothing else, but to transform them into positive. Hence, each disease is due to an excess of negative energies. If you cannot turn them into positive, find a vent, from where the excess to flow out. The negative energy in the organism is an invited guest, of which you shall get rid.

When the energies of the human organism strive to the center of the Earth, it gets ill. In order to recover, these energies shall turn to the center of the Sun.

If man's doppelganger goes out and comes in normally, the stomach works well; the brain is in good shape, and man is healthy. Most of the indispositions are due to an anomaly in the brain. That is why your first task is to regulate the brain energies so that they to flow properly. Put your hand often over the head or run your fingers through the hair from up to down in the way you comb.

Many diseases are due to tension, caused by the natural electricity or by the magnetism on certain organs. For example, somebody complains of headache, of heartache, or of lung aches. These aches are due to the pressure, which the atmospheric electricity exerts on these organs. One shall know in what way to transform the excessive energies in his organism. Sometimes magnetism in human organism is more than it is needed, as a result of which he experiences certain painful states. By studying his organism, one comes to a position to understand that many of his painful states are due to atmospheric influences.

When water decreases, human life decreases, too. The changes, which happen on the Earth, happen also with the human body. A big part of the body is water. Many people suffer of lack of water in the organism. Water is the reason for the warmth of organism.

The lack of water cools the organism. On the other hand, too much water heats it up.

Lack of water in the organism makes one nervous and dry. He begins to annoy, becomes sharp and ready to be angry and arguing with everyone. How nervousness can be influenced? Through hot water. Take a glass of hot water and drink spoon by spoon. During that time watch after which spoon you will get calm. If you do not have hot water, you can make the experiment with cold water.

When in the organism gathers much water, which cannot be assimilated, it produces many diseases: dropsy, pleurisy and others.

It is noticed that some diseases are caused by an excess quantity of water in the body. To get rid of the excess water, doctors put one under such conditions, at such heat, at which the excess water to evaporate. If iron is in excess, the human body needs to be put in such mental conditions, in which iron melts and evaporates.

Constipation is due to deficiency of water in the blood. Chestache - deficiency of warmth in feelings. When human feelings are warm, legs, hands and his whole body is warm, as a result of which he feels in good spirits.

All diseases are caused by disharmony between the sympathetic and brain systems.

I say: Is the nervous system the one, which is upset? It is not upset, but blocked. I have a stomachache. Why? Those nerves of the spinal cord, through which the energy goes to the stomach and abdomen, are blocked. Expose your backbone to Sun, in order your nerves to unblock. If they do not unblock, the pains will inevitably follow you. Diseases are due to deficiency of energy. Blockages occur not only in the physical body, but in the other bodies, too.

The power, contained in the nitrogen, is associated with the nervous system and brain. Therefore, when nitrogen begins to decrease, anxiety is born in people. The fact that some people get mad or are seized by apoplexy is due to the lack of nitrogen – of its powers in brain substance, blood circulation is not proper, more blood comes to the head, which cannot be withdrawn back and it blocks certain centers, causing a strike and these blocked centers or organs are paralyzed.

Diseases, which attack people, are due to past and present sins. Nothing remains unpunished. Microbes that plague human organism today are nothing else, but the poison of fear, of hatred that cattle, chickens, lambs have felt toward man when he killed them. Is this possible? It is possible. In the way an insulting word may poison and destroy the human organism, in the same way fear and hatred of animals, which man kills, poison his organism.

Know that microbes, which stack in human organism, are those, to which he has a certain predisposition. They become partners with him and begin to draw on his energy. Imperceptibly, he gets ill and becomes a victim. It is impossible for a microbe, with which you are in a disagreement, to stack into you.

The greater the quantity of gold in the blood is, the more healthy one is. Diseases are due to insufficient quantity of gold in the blood of people. To increase this gold, one shall lead a clean and noble life. Gold is a symbol of the Sun, of the energy, of the health, of purity.

Many diseases are caused by lack of organic gold in the blood. Weakness and anemia are due to insufficient quantity of iron in the blood. When the human mind is still, it shows that he has less phosphorus in his blood.

If iron is predominant in the blood, it produces a kind of thoughts, if copper predominates – another kind of thoughts. In general, each element - iron, copper, tin, lead, silver, gold - produces a specific effect on the thoughts and feelings of people.

Any disorder in the physical body, either in its sympathetic system or in its nervous one, shows that there is a lack of an element in the blood. This element is provided not only by food, but by thoughts and feelings.

If you have a look at the hand of man, as a clairvoyant, around it, you will notice a light, mobile hand, which is a doppelganger of the physical one. As long as the doppelganger of the human hand acts correctly, the physical hand is normal. If the doppelganger is crippled somehow, the physical hand will be crippled, too. Not only the hand, but the whole human body has a specific doppelganger. If the doppelganger separates prematurely from the physical man totally or partially, various mutilations, diseases, etc. appear. The total or partial paralysis is due to premature separation of the doppelganger from the physical body of somebody. The premature separation of the doppelganger is due to incorrect adoption of the natural energies through the hands and feet.

The main reason of diseases is due to the disharmony between the doppelganger and the physical body. In the front part of the brain there are a particular kind of brain white threads, through which the activity of human consciousness, which is related to the doppelganger, manifests. The doppelganger is a device, by which the powers of nature manifest. The physical body lives thanks to its doppelganger and if the relationship between the body and the doppelganger are not correct and harmonious, lots of diseases occur.

If someone faints, you shall know that the relation between the doppelganger and the body has lost for a moment, the connection has been broken.

Sufferings, especially with spiritual people, are due to their great sensitiveness, to the fact that the ether, astral doppelganger goes out more than it is needed, as a result of which it receives more impressions and, of course, suffers more.

The whole man's body, outside and inside, is wrapped with a special matter, called matrix. When the matrix is healthy, one feels well. He is in good spirits, healthy and strong. If the matrix cracks, lots of chemical processes happen in the human body, which affect it painfully. As long as one keeps unnatural thoughts and feelings or if he doubts, suspects, speaks evil, his matrix may always crack.

Many of the human painful states and bad spirits are due to the shrinking of capillaries. The shrinking and expansion of capillaries happens under the influence of electricity and magnetism. One should live a normal life, respect the laws of nature, in order great shrinking of the capillaries not to happen.

What kind of thoughts and feelings cause shrinking of the capillaries? Negative ones. So, every evil thought, every bad feeling, and every bad deed narrows the capillaries and interrupts the flows of electricity and magnetism in the human organism. Electricity and magnetism move along certain lines. They have a specific rhythm. When the lines of movement and rhythm change, certain disharmony establishes in the organism and we say that somebody is ill.

Aim at harmonious movements of the eyes, hands, and of the whole body. Beware of disharmonious movements as of unnatural and alien ones. Beware of imitations. Disharmonious movements upset the organism in the same way, in which bad and spoilt food does.

Watch small children up to the age of 6 or 7. Their movements are quite correct, natural, but between the ages of 7 and 14, their movements become artificial. They cause various diseases.

Man does not know how to walk properly yet. While walking, he shakes, as a result of which a concussion occurs in the spinal cord. This concussion is transferred to the brain, and from there, to the entire nervous system. After all that, people are wondering why they are nervous.

Eyes weaken when one does not make the needed exercises. Many people do not watch as they should. They open their eyes widely. They stare, but it is not watching. It is correct, when you want to see something, not to spin your head to one side and to another, but to move your eyes. You shall move your eyes up, down, sideways, in the direction, where the observed object is.

The reason of cold is poor breathing. Whoever catches a cold, he should know that there is a deviation in his breathing – the breathing is not rhythmic, as a result of which not enough quantity of air is received. When breathing improves, the cold will disappear. Nature warns one through cold that he shall work. If you disregard that warning, it sends him fever.

Someone complains that he cannot breathe freely and that his heart does not beat normally. He calls doctors, drinks drugs, but nothing helps. The reason is in the diaphragm. It has raised and presses the stomach, the lungs and heart and the entire organism suffers in this way. Therefore, breathe deeply in order your lungs to be filled up with air and the diaphragm to adjust.

You suffer because you are not in harmony with colors.

Which is the reason for diseases? The absence of a color in man. If he lacks the red color of love, the yellow color of wisdom or the blue color of truth, he will by no means be ailing. Therefore, in order not to be ailing, you have to introduce these colors both in your organisms and your psyches, i.e. in your sensual and mental lives.

The science of the future humanity, which is the science of the sixth race, will begin exactly with the law of coordination. Every organ in man must be coordinated with all other organs.

In accordance with the law of coordination it is determined man to cover 2-3-5-10 km per day. If he is scared and does not accomplish what nature has determined to him, it will not be long before it imposes a fine for failure in obeying its laws. In addition, nature has determined man to eat clean and simple food. Furthermore, it is determined how many times per minute man has to breathe. Some people take in air promiscuously, breathe unevenly, as a result of which there is no coordination between the other organs, either. If there is no complete coordination between all organs, lots of painful states will occur.

Diagnostics

Each line of a hand, every feature of a face, each center of a head are letters, showing one's life and work from the distant past to the present.

It is a mastery to determine the diagnosis 10 years before the occurrence of a disease in order one to be able to take measures in advance. This can be done only by a doctor, who knows the occult sciences. Before becoming fat, you shall tell that person what to do.

These studies, which are not recognized nowadays here, will solve the issues in the future. You will study these studies more carefully - palmistry, phrenology, physiognomy, graphology, Kabbalah and all their subdivisions.

If contemporary doctors knew these sciences, there should not be a reason for opening one's brain or stomach to determine the diagnosis of a disease, but only through a glance at the eyes or hands, at the nails or at the horoscope, they should determine not only the disease, but also the reasons for it.

Before getting ill, you can help yourself to avoid certain states, which expect you. For this purpose, make your own measurements to determine your diagnosis while you are still healthy.

Both drinking and eating are processes not only of the physical, but also of the mental and heart worlds. One will suffer in the world, in which he overeats.

There is a certain relation between the organs. For example, the width of the nose underneath and the temporal zones show the evolution of the vital (phlegmatic) temperament. Furthermore, the width of the nose is related to the width of the hand, as well as to the width of the face. The structure of the stomach is in relation to the structure of the fingers. One, who understands the law of the relation, may determine the state of one organ through another one.

If you make a mistake, you will feel pain either in the stomach or in the lungs, or in the legs, or in the fingers, or in the backbone, or in the liver ... The localization of the disease in the various places shows what kind of a mistake you have made.

Any violation of the laws of the physical world produces an upset in the stomach, abdomen and intestines; any violation of the spiritual laws - in the lungs, feelings; any violation of the laws in the mental world produces disorder in the head.

Looking at your eyes, I think of your truth. Looking at your ears, I think of your wisdom. Looking at your mouth, I think of your love. Looking at your hands, I think of your justice, with which you work. Looking your feet, I think of your virtues.

It is enough to look at the hand of anybody to guess how long he will live on the Earth. This is determined by the lines of the hand, as well as by their length and width. In addition, the wider the nose is and more opened the nostrils are, the longer one's life is, he receives more air, and the less air one receives, the less his blood is oxidized, because of which diseases come frequently and more carbonic acid, more sediments are released.

If one has very thin lips, it means that he has repressed his feelings, that he cannot give much. This man does not like to eat much, either. He does not pamper himself.

The cells, which form the two lips, are rational. Do not keep them very tight nor relaxed, opened. They shall be barely closed and free. The same concerns the eyes. Do not look at dreadful things and ugly images. Never watch how animals are slaughtered or how crime is being committed.

If you examine under a magnifying glass the nervous system or the eyes of a man, who has views of the Old Testament, as well as of a man with beliefs of the New Testament, you will see what a difference there is in their structure. Past, present and future of a man may be recognized by his eyes. Everything that may happen to someone is written in his eyes. If someone is suffering of consumption, or no matter what disease, there are signs in his eyes that speak of that disease.

The change in the eye color depends on the change in the mental state. In fact, this change is due to weakening of the vibrations of the human brain. This weakening of the vibrations affects the brightness of the eyes, due to which they change their color. The eye color serves as a diagnosis for determining the mental state of a person and the state of his mind. The eyes are a mirror of one's inner life.

Sometimes spots appear in the human eyes like the spots on the Sun. Man's eye may be divided into 12 circles, which represent the 12 signs of the zodiac in movement. Like the sunspots, which are the reason for accidents and sufferings on the Earth, the spots in the human eyes are the reasons for lots of painful states. Spots and blurs, which appear in the eyes, predict a disease that may occur in 10 or 20 years. One, who understands the science of the eyes, may prevent him from that disease.

If I look at your ear, I can guess by it how many years you are going to live, what kind of diseases you are going to suffer of and from what you will die. I can guess the same by the nail – all diseases may be guessed. It is a written book.

There are doctors, who determine the diagnosis of the patient by his hand and nails. They guess not only the current condition of the patient, but also what expects him in the future. Before someone gets ill, spots appear at some places of the hand and nails. This shows that there are no secrets in the world.

If you want to know if a disease expects you, or any state of illness, watch your nails. If a white spot appears on any of your nails, you shall know that you are going to pass through a disease. And if the spots appear at your left hand, they have one meaning; if they appear at your right hand, they have another meaning. In general, the least white spot on a nail is a sign of a painful state.

White spots on nails indicate great stress of the nervous system, leading to disease. If you notice a white spot on any of your nails, take measures immediately: introduce into your mind a great, higher idea, which calms the nervous system. These spots appear also when there are big emotional shocks. There is nothing bad in the appearance of white spots. They are warning signs, which make you take measures against the painful state, which is to come.

White spots on nails indicate abnormality in the nervous system. White spots on nails are similar to the spots of the Sun. The more spots the Sun has, the more energy, the more abundance exists in nature. The same happens with a person who has white spots on the nails. He is extremely active, releases more energy from himself, as a result of which he extremely exhausts. To get rid of these spots, one shall focus his mind on a certain thought. For a period of 2-3 months, he may remove the spots from his nails.

If you have a headache, you shall know that your stomach is a mess - they are related. The methods for treating them are so simple that each of you may apply them.

If the neck is very wide – more than 35 cm to 41-42 cm, that person is exposed to apoplexy. He must do something to reduce the thickness of his neck. The neck of one, who is 165 cm tall, must be no more than 35 cm wide. If the width is reduced and it reaches to 29-30 cm, one is exposed to other risks. He shall eat better to increase the thickness of his neck.

If you look at one's face on both sides, at the cheek-bones, you will understand what the state of the stomach is. If the face under the cheek-bones is sunken, the stomach is weak.

To understand what the state of your liver is, look at the color of your face, the light in your eyes and their vitality. These things add beauty to the face.

When the liver is functioning properly, one's face has a pleasant pink color.

The nose of nervous people begins to sharpen gradually, and this should not happen. One should have a sharp and alert mind, but not a sharp nose.

One of the simplest ways for determining the length of one's life is the following: put a finger on the top of the skin and press a little; if a dimple remains there, he will not live long, but if the dimple disappears quickly, he has energy, and will live long.

One, who has more iron in his blood, is irritable, quick-tempered. Suspicious people have more lead. One, who has not stable emotions, has more copper. Only the presence of gold does not cause sufferings for now, but one wants to have more and more, to store up. All elements exist disproportionally distributed in the human blood, in the nervous system and in the cells, and exactly this disproportion leads to a number of dissonances. Therefore, one should know how to renovate himself in order to neutralize the harmful effects of the elements in his organism.

If a person has an idealistic impulse in his life, he walks upright. Once he becomes a materialist, he starts to bend toward the ground. When he loses faith in himself and his fellows, he begins to stoop. If one stoops, this shows that there is a defect in the mind. The backbone is a perpendicular. Any deviation and any stoop indicate a distortion in the character.

A good man is wrapped in a magnificent garment that does not let cold. If your feet are used to get cold, good is weak in you. If your hands are used to get cold, justice is weak. If your eyes do not see well – you have breached the truth somewhere. If your ears do not hear well, you have breached the wisdom.

If you have a diamond with you and it darkens, this means that you are ill. Stones are infected by humans.

One may read not only by the lines of the face, but also by the colors that surround somebody. This may be done by a clairvoyant, but not by a normal person.

The stronger, more spiritual, and more raised one is, the whiter, sparkling and more pleasant the aura, which comes out of him, is. If a person gets ill, the aura darkens. Darkening may become partially or entirely. Each ill part is dark. It is necessary one to restore the light of the head or of the stomach or of the ill organ. This will also happen if he strengthens his mind and raises his vibrations.

If the hands are wet, it means that your feelings are not in a natural position. If they are dry – the mind is not in a natural position.

Celestial Objects and Health

Today planets are considered as symbols, but in the future people will reach higher development. They will understand their essence, will find out what secrets are hidden in them. Planets are living rational creatures, with whom one is directly connected, but he does not know it, nor has knowledge of the creatures inhabiting these planets.

All planets are transformers of the Divine energy in the various organisms. All the planets are inhabited by rational creatures. The Jupetarians have dignity, a sense of themselves. They are proud, but merciful. The Saturnians are philosophers, deep, suspicious; they always criticize, and are in doubt. They are the most ancient inhabitants of the Solar system, but Uranus and Neptune have originated before Saturn - their inhabitants are more ancient than those of Saturn.

Respiratory, stomach and nervous systems are created under different conditions and times under the influence of the planets. The same concerns the body parts. For example, arms are under the influence of Gemini and Mercury. Legs - under the influence of Pisces and Jupiter. Lungs - under the influence of Cancer, and the head - under the influence of Aries.

Modern people need to study the dynamics of the human body in relation to the planetary influences on it. In this way, one will understand that certain body cells are under the influence of the Sun, others - under the influence of Sirius, third ones - under the influence of Jupiter, etc. In general, the higher creatures and planets are connected to a person, the higher and more developed the matter of his body is. The more developed the matter of human body is, the higher one's life. The level of human development is determined by the matter of his organism. Human life manifests through the matter. The more developed the mind of man is, the more connected to the stars and planets one is. When one uses the influence of all suns in the Cosmos, man attains perfection.

There is only one sun in the human brain, around which all planets move. Whatever you see in the sky, it is the same in the brain. What we call movement of powers, of power centers in the brain, is nothing else, but the effect of the outer planets on the brain.

Almost all planets have points in the human cerebrum.

Jupiter is in the middle of the crown of the head; Saturn is alongside in the upper part of the head; Venus - in the upper part, in the middle of the forehead and nape.

Mars is on both sides of the head, above the ears. Jupiter gives length and activity to the head. Saturn gives extension to the human mind, to consciousness. The Moon gives extension to the forehead. Mars also gives extension. All planets affect the brain. Earth and all stars affect the brain, too.

The powers of the Sun organize your heart and lungs.

The powers of Saturn organize the liver and the bones.

The powers of Mars – the gall and the reproductive organs.

The powers of Jupiter – the stomach and solar plexus.

The powers of Venus – the kidneys.

The powers of Mercury and the Moon – the brain and nerves. The Moon also affects the female reproductive organs. The spleen is a conductor of the solar energy and is under the influence of the Sun. Jupiter rules the thymus gland.

Mercury – the thyroid gland.

Saturn and Uranus – the pituitary.

Neptune – the pineal.

The Sun affects mainly the solar plexus and the sympathetic nervous system. To coordinate the powers of his organism, one must connect his sympathetic nervous system to brain one, as well as the bone system to the muscle one. When one cannot give a proper expression of the spiritual powers within himself, he will roughen.

One's task includes harmonizing of the powers of the organism and establishment of proper relations with all stars. The modern person does not perceive correctly the energies of the Cosmos, as a result of which more energies, than it is needed, are accumulated in certain places in the organism, while in others - less. This improper allocation of the energies in the human organism causes his misfortunes and sufferings, his discontents. Even the most sublime energies, stored in one place, cause a painful state.

When one gets ill, one shall connect with the energy of the Sun and the Moon. If you cannot connect directly with them, use those plants and minerals, which are connected with the energies of the Sun and the Moon and transform them properly.

Under the influence of the Sun, the cosmic consciousness in man awakens. The Sun is what awakens the human mind. The Sun is alive, collective creature that has cosmic consciousness. Mind is in it. When that cosmic, Divine consciousness awakens in man, the Sun begins to think about him and then one is healthy and lives long.

The milfoil is related to the physical sun, and the Sun is from what we get regenerating energy in our whole nature. The Spirit of God gives energy to the Sun and it introduces it into the cerebrum, in the larynx, in the heart, in the soul. The milfoil has derived some its colors from Sirius and Orion.

The milfoil is the celestial beauty with all planets and all colors. It contains thousands of centers only in the cerebrum and these centers distribute the thousands of colors that give an incredible shine - the most beautiful shine. The Sun is an expression of the milfoil, which is ruled by the Spirit of God.

Planets relate to certain elements, especially metals. The Moon is related to silver; the Sun – to gold; Mars - to iron. If a person suffers from a deficiency of one of these elements in his blood, he gets ill. In order his state to be improved, that element must be introduced in his blood. In general, any disorder in one's physical body, either in the sympathetic or in the nervous system, shows a lack of an element in his blood. Once the necessary quantity of the relevant element is provided, the state of the organism improves. The lack of any element in the blood is provided not only from food, but also through our thoughts and feelings. There are occasions when the organism feels the need of certain thoughts and feelings. They must, by no means, enter into the mind and heart of man. Knowing this, you should apply astrology also through self-education for building up the nervous system. Then, through your thoughts and feelings, you will introduce into your blood all the elements, of which shortage is felt. This is a science that must be studied not only theoretically, but also practically. This knowledge is not acquired at once, but gradually.

Cherry is under the influence of Venus. The same concerns the apple. Plants and fruits contain such a kind of energy, depending on the planets, to which they are connected. On the other side, planets are connected with the stars of the zodiac. If you want to influence in any way your character, you shall use such food, which gives you the relevant energies. In the future, man will eat the food, which corresponds to the relevant planets, ruling on that day. On Monday you will eat food that is under the influence of the Moon; on Tuesday - which is under the influence of Mars, etc.

Knowing the influence of planets on humans, especially of the Sun, you must have the right attitude towards it. If one is in harmony with the Sun, he will be in harmony with the Moon and Earth. The good effect of the Sun on humans improves the state of the arterial blood. The relationship between the Sun's influence on arterial blood hides in the harmony between thoughts and feelings of people. The Sun raises human thoughts and feelings, due to which human blood purifies. And vice versa – one's harmonious thoughts, feelings and deeds are in harmony with the energies of the Sun, Moon and Earth, as a result of which one enjoys life and benefits of its goods.

Any blocking of feelings introduces a certain anomaly in the functions of the heart, resulting in change in the pulse. To restore the normal activity of the heart, one must enter into harmony with Nature, connect his heart with the common pulse of the Cosmic heart. Each planetary system also has its own heart, which is connected to the common Cosmic heart. The heart of our Solar system is the Sun. The rhythmic movement of blood in the human heart is determined by the rhythmic waves of the Sun. For 10 days, make the following experience: three times per day (in the morning, at noon and in the evening), every day, absorb deeply in yourself and say: "I want my heart to beat rhythmically, to merge with the pulse of the Sun and send properly its energy all over the world."

Young people have not yet built those spiritual organs, which are favorably influenced by Saturn, Uranus and Mercury. Having not developed yet their spiritual organs, when they find themselves under the influence of these planets, young people use their spiritual powers for physical needs. As a result of the above they roughen. When one cannot give a proper expression of the spiritual powers within himself, he will surely roughen. It is impossible to have spiritual achievements by physical efforts.

One, who wants to be born on Earth, shall know astrology very well. He shall know in which year to be born, in which month, on which day, hour, minute and second. If you were not born in the year, month, week, day, hour, minute, and second, when you had to be born, your works on Earth will not go well. It is not because Nature is unwilling to help you, but there is a discrepancy between the choice of time when you have come and the natural and planetary influence.

When a patient wants to be cured of his illness, he shall watch the Moon, when it empties, and connect with it. If the Moon fills, he must close the shutters on the windows, in order its light not to enter his room. If we talk about the sunlight, both ill and healthy people shall expose to its beneficial effect.

If a child becomes ill during the emptying of the Moon, it will surely get better. If a child gets ill during the time when the Sun goes to the southern hemisphere - from 22nd September onwards, it will surely get better. Even in these favorable conditions for recovery of the child, his mother may complicate his state and send him prematurely to the other world by her negative thoughts.

Aging

One of the tasks of modern man is to prolong his life.

After the Fall, man has shortened his life. He needs to work on himself to prolong his life and return in his initial state. Therefore, if one wants to prolong his life, he has to lead a simple and clean life, without any alien influences and external impurities. If you meet such a person, you will see that his life is simple, modest: in food, in clothing, in relationships.

Is it natural for one to get older? It is not natural. One gets older for the sole reason that he does not obey that balance, which he has to have in his mind.

Aging is the most terrible pathology. Thoughts of aging are microbes. When people get ill of these microbes, they get older. They are like termites. They eat everything sacred in man, leaving only bones.

People of feelings get older faster than people of sober thought.

Life length depends on the proper relationship that one has with the First Cause, his fellow, and himself. Man determines the line if his life by himself – whether it will be short or long. By studying the law of heredity, you will see that entire clans follow the life of short lines, and others – the life of long lines.

Children, born to parents, who come from the clan of long lines, will live a long life, and vice versa.

For now, man is determined to live 120 years on Earth, If he takes off earlier the old and dirty clothes, we say that he has left Earth earlier.

From the age of 50 to 120, work is the most useful and productive. It is the work for your raising and the raising of the entire mankind.

One, who hates, becomes more energetic, more courageous, more arrogant, as a result of which his muscles stiffen, his face becomes rough and raw. One, who loves, looks mild and weak, but his life prolongs, his body is plastic, and his muscles - flexible.

When the Sun much influences somebody (it means that it is well aspected in a horoscope), then he lives long.

As long as I think of myself without love, I am getting older. When I think of oxen, of the house, of my wife without love, I am getting older. When I think of my child without love, I am getting older.

Sorrows prolong life. Without sorrows and sufferings, human life would be heavier and shorter than it is now. The more mentally developed humanity is, the greater its sufferings are.

One, who welcomes suffering with joy, will live long. A young man, who remains true to his love, will live long. Someone, who does not mix food, will live long.

If you know how to suffer, you will rejuvenate. As you avoid sufferings and do not evaluate them, you are aging. If one does not evaluate his joy either, he is aging.

You have become older, because you do not accept all good that passes through you.

The length of life depends on the amount of air you take into your lungs. Apart from that there is a rhythm in Nature, a pulse that supports life. The occasional improper pulse of the heart or the very slow pulse or the very quick pulse depends on this common Cosmic pulse.

Mistakes make you older. One makes himself older by the way of eating, by lots of emotions, by anxious thoughts, by rotten, stale food.

Aging, with regard to the body, is aging, but it is rejuvenation in terms of human mind.

Old age is a law of rejuvenation.

If you hate someone, you shorten your life, but if you go to reconcile, you will continue your life. If you reconcile, if you come to love everybody, whom you have hated by now, if you make all needed sacrifices, you will live long. Anyone, who hates his father, will not live long.

Once you start to get irritated of little things, you have already entered in the old age. In order not to get older, do not get irritated.

When one starts to chat too much, he gets older. If he is not satisfied and is on bad terms with the world, he gets older much quicker.

People age of ignorance and worries.

If you want to get older quicker, complain.

If the tongue is getting white, you are getting older. If the tongue is getting red, you are rejuvenating. White tongue indicates that digestion is not normal. After this try to improve your stomach in order your tongue to improve.

When the solar, brain and sympathetic systems do not function properly, blackness under the eyes appears, or this happens also if the liver is more excited than it should be. The liver is an enterprise of Nature, where all lower feelings are created. The animal conditions that animals have are due to the liver. Our indisposition is due to the liver. It shall function properly. It has two functions, two services. It helps digestion and these animal feelings are due to it. He is near, adjacent to the stomach brain or to the solar plexus.

Very often old people suffer from not cleaned blood and this is the cause of blood pressure. Blood pressure is the venous blood, which collects in the veins and blood circulation is not proper.

Such people get older prematurely. The less venous blood, the better. The less bad thoughts, the better. Good thoughts are the arterial blood.

One, who wants to prolong his life, shall refrain. From what? First of all from too much eating. You shall always remain a little bit hungry, not eat enough. So, a little stock of unused energy remains in the organism and it renovates it. If you overeat, you are shortening your life. Moreover, man shall be pleased with what he eats. So, contentment prolongs life. You shall never overeat and you shall always eat with gratitude and contentment – these are the two rules for prolonging of life.

As long as good meals attract you, you are on the path of death.

Two things prolong life: rational eating, i.e. obeying of a certain diet and normal sufferings. By not overeating and by not eating enough, one prolongs his life.

One, who eats without chewing, shortens his life.

One, who eats quickly, dies early. You shall chew well on both sides of the teeth - on the right and on the left. When you are not well and sick, do not eat. If you are angry, do not eat. Wait until everything in you calms down.

In order to live longer, you need to understand the life of the plants and know how to use their nectar.

Music and songs have a good effect on human psyche. One, who wants to live a long time, shall sing.

Love renovates the life of the cells.

Rejuvenation is an internal psychic process. There is a special kind of glands in the brain and in the sympathetic nervous system, which humans do not know yet how to manipulate.

Modern scientists do not know yet what the roles of these glands are. One day, when they understand their roles, they will be able to use them consciously as a means of rejuvenation.

One can rejuvenate not only by an alchemical way, but by his mind, too. Man's bright thought creates round him a pleasant atmosphere, which makes him able to perceive what is nice and beautiful from the living Nature.

One is young if he is ready at any moment to oblige anyone, who is in need. One is young if he bears all hardships and sufferings with joy, studies, does not lie, is fearless, works, and is faultless in each respect.

You eat bread, without thinking about its attitude toward your will; drink water without being aware of the attitude - toward life, as well as toward your heart. While drinking water and cooling yourself down, say in yourself: "In the way water cools, let, in the same way, my feelings cool down and refresh the tired and thirsty traveler." If you pronounce these words every day, your heart will renovate. This is one of the methods, which Nature uses for rejuvenating humans and raising their spirits.

Retain neither yours, nor somebody else's mistakes in your mind - this is a method for rejuvenation.

Do not hold somebody else's mistakes in yourself for a long time, because you will catch the same mistakes.

One gets younger while he is smiling. One, who studies God's truth, does not get older.

If you can read the Old and New Testaments 99 times, you will rejuvenate.

There are lots of ways for rejuvenating. Stand up early in the morning, grab the lobe of the ear. Then massage the bone behind the ear. Do this every morning.

Fasting is used for renovating of the body. It is a method of rejuvenation. After the fasting, eat as long as it is possible uniform food, which requires less effort for digestion, in order appetite not to be stirred, in order lungs to be able to develop and you to take in more prana from the air and water and take out more juices from food than now.

If you want to rejuvenate, make the following experiment. If you are at the age of 50 or 60, every night when you go to bed, say to yourself that tomorrow you will be 5 years younger than you are today. Make this experiment for a week. If you have managed to put that thought in your subconscious, at the end of the week, you will really be 5 years younger. Do so for several weeks until you get younger and even reach the age of 25.

In the course of 5 years at most one can rejuvenate. To achieve this, he must make the following experiment: every night, when he goes to bed, let him say that in the morning he will find a black hair on his head. On the next day he shall do the same. And indeed, every morning he is going to find one black hair more. Day after day his hairs will get black, until one morning, when he will see that his whole hair has become black. This depends on the strength of his mind and his faith.

Love is the one that supports life. If one loses Love, he is slowly dying.

People die from lovelessness. If there is no one to love somebody, he soon dies.

Dying is nothing else, but taking off old clothes and dressing of new ones. It is impossible for somebody always to have new and good clothing, which is always clean.

If one loses half of his weight, dies. When the balance between the powers of the heart and the powers of mind is broken, then death comes.

Death is a tax-gatherer, who serves the karmic spirits. These spirits are also called guards. They are present at anyone's dying and argue on his soul.

It is defined for everybody from what he will die and when he will die.

When a man dies, he leaves everything on Earth. The only thing, which he takes with him, is the capital deposited in his brain. When a person is dying, his soul stays next to his head, waiting for his last breath, in order to take this capital immediately.

During the entire life it has been working on it, has been turning the lower into higher, has organized it and now it comes down to take it. It takes only the essence of the brain.

TREATMENT

Treatment in General

There is something in human nature that needs internal stirring. And every pain and every test is for strengthening of your spiritual nature. If you do not have tests, you will not develop.

There are several ways for treatment of patients. One of the ways is natural healing. Leave the patient to Nature. It will not be long before he recovers. This method is the best. The second way is treatment by a doctor. A doctor will come. He will recommend a medicine and after a while the patient gets better. But there is also a third way of treatment – the Divine one. The patient recovers immediately through it.

In order one to be healthy, he must rely on himself and the direct contact with Nature. Nature will help more than people. The first condition: trust in God, trust in Nature, trust in yourself and finally - in the others.

The most powerful medicine is light. The most powerful medicine is air – the breath of God. The most powerful medicine is the bread - the word of God. These drugs are also used by plants. The healing properties of plants are due to light, air, water and food, which they perceive. If future doctors perceive my system of healing, there will be good results. One doctor will be a conductor of the light, another - of the air, third ones – of the water, and the fourth ones – of the food. If one is not as sweet as fruits, as mild as water, as movable as air and light, he can gain nothing. God has entered into bread, fruits, water, air and light – He has sacrificed Himself. One, who loves God, perceives Him as a part of himself. Such a person gets treatment. So, eat with love, drink with love, and take in light with love.

One has four points of contact with God - by light, by air, by water and by food.

Remember this definition: one must love himself, in order to treat his body. One must love his fellow to treat his heart. One, who wants to succeed in everything, to bless himself, he shall love God. There are benefits only in love toward God.

One day, when they know the laws of light and warmth, people will cure all diseases by light and warmth. Incurable diseases will not remain.

If you investigate the state of a patient, you will see that three factors are involved in his recovering: Nature, a doctor and the patient himself. 50% of the help comes from Nature, 25% - from the doctor and 25% - from the patient. The patient is responsible for the last word. If he does not take part in his treatment, the help of Nature and the doctor will be in vain.

It is not easy to treat people. You treat someone in some way, but instead of improvement, his state worsens. In general, it is impossible all people to be treated with the same remedy. For each disease, for each person, a specific remedy is needed. There are as many remedies as many people there are in the world. Therefore, if one wants to be treated properly and together with that to help his fellow, he must study that science, which reveals the secrets of Nature.

When some people ask me, if we shall call doctors for a disease, I say: that issue is already solved. If you follow the laws of the old culture, call doctors, but if you follow the laws of the occult school, do not call doctors. Doctors will heal the world, but, for an occult student, the disease is not something accidental. It has its purpose. For himself, for his soul, everyone will look for his internal doctor.

It is difficult indeed for one to transfer a thought from one place to another in its essence. For example, when one gets ill, he calls a doctor. If the doctor manages to transfer the thought of the patient from his head to another place, he can immediately recover. If he cannot do that, he shall use one of the two methods – homeopathic - with low doses or allopathic - with heavy doses. There is also another way for treatment: leaving the disease to come to its crisis and coming down to begin from there – i.e. the disappearance. Each person has hidden powers, which have to be awakened. If you can wake up these powers, the state of the patient improves naturally. If the hidden powers in the organism cannot wake up naturally: by sweating, by tours, by bathes, doctors resort to drugs in small or in large doses. There are occasions when the doctor gives medications in a larger dose than it is needed, and instead of evoking the activity of the hidden powers, he stops them.

In medicine, there are two theories: allopathy – for maximum doses and homeopathy - for small doses. For example, at allopathy, you may take the drugs from an entire pharmacy without experiencing any disruption in the organism, without any specific reaction. At small doses, you may have a greater result. The following is a law: at small efforts you have the same results as with large ones.

Small quantities produce greater results than larger ones. Homeopathy uses extremely small quantities - treat in a homeopathic way. An extremely small number of the kilogram of a given substance, unit of measurement with 60 zeros at the end, may produce a great effect on the human organism. It is enough for the patient to take just one drop of this extremely watered matter and he will immediately recover. Divine energy is put in this drop. If you believe in the power of this energy, you will recover in two or three days.

Today we cannot utilize all occult methods, because there are such occult methods, which, if applied, do you know what will happen? Your organism, your brain, your muscular system, your arterial system, your nervous system will not endure, they are not adapted. Hindus have special methods, which they apply, but they have practiced them for thousands of years. For example, one of these methods is the method of deep breathing that Western nations cannot use. However, these methods are artificial. We have other natural methods. White Brotherhood use these natural methods, which are excellent.

There 7-8 methods of healing for each person. One may be treated in a spiritual way only sometimes. Few people can be treated in a spiritual way. Which people? Only those in whom there is absolutely no doubt. They should have full confidence in you, and you shall be totally honest with them. If that confidence and honesty do not exist between them, no spiritual healing may happen. Then you have to apply one of the methods of Nature: water, herbs, etc. Besides this method of healing, there is a third method. It is music.

In recent times, in almost all European countries, there are clinics that implement electricity and magnetism as methods of treatment. Through these methods they want to awaken the respective powers of the organism, which raise its vibration in man, too.

When the vibrations of the organism raise, one recovers. In this way, even the most hardly treated diseases like cancer, tuberculosis and others, are treated. At this treatment, the patient goes through major crises. But if he passes through the crises, his state improves. If he withstands the first crisis, the last ones pass easily. They gradually weaken until they finally stop and the patient recovers. By crises, the organism cleans from the harmful and toxic elements in it.

To recover, a patient should clean his blood. He himself should undertake that task. How? By breathing of fresh air, by exposing his back to sun and by eating of clean, healthy food. There are other methods for purifying the blood. It depends on man what methods he will apply to purify his blood not in months or years, but in one day. Usually one uses one or another method in accordance with his mind.

The mind knows the causes of diseases, but cannot cure them. Soul cures the diseases. It is enough it to wish to cure a disease in order the desired to be achieved.

True doctor may expel a disease out from a patient through some formulas or words. The doctor can chase out spirits.

One may heal himself when the reserve vital energy awakes in him and is pushed to activity. If you want to treat yourself in a natural way, use mainly the months April and May, when Nature is rich in vital energy. Every day of those months worths millions of dollars. What one gains at that time of the year, he cannot gain the same within another period.

Things are strictly mathematically defined in the world. There is time for sowing, and there is time designated for treatment. This is the Divine principle.

It is not easy to handle with ill people. The most discontent people in the world are ill people. Why? They expect everything from the doctor. If he does not help them, they are dissatisfied with him. To avoid discontentment of patients, a doctor shall know whom to treat and whom not. If the bones behind the ears of a patient are protuberant, he may be treated. He withstands diseases. If the patient's chin is wide and the lower jaw is a bit protuberant, that person may be treated.

There are two ways of healing: natural and immediate - Divine. You can not heal a sinner immediately, but a righteous man may be immediately healed no matter what his disease is.

Contemporary people treat only the physical body, because they partly know only it. Apostles and Disciples of Christ speak also of a spiritual body. Wise men and great masters speak of seven bodies, in which one lives. Humans have already begun to live also in their spiritual bodies, but they are not aware of the other bodies.

If a person falls ill physically, the disease affects also the spiritual body, and vice versa. If one wants to heal himself, he has to get in touch with his spiritual body. If he heals just in a physical way, he will achieve nothing. At nights, while sleeping, man leaves his physical body and during that time complete purification and renewal of cells takes place. When he gets purified, he enters back in it and wakes up. If you sleep well, your body cleans well and you wake up in good spirits and renovated.

You may treat yourself, but if from above, from the invisible world, light beings do not participate, you can never recover. Remedy is just a conductor.

When you get ill, first turn to God, then to your soul and finally to the doctor. You walk in the opposite direction and that is why you fail.

If a person can be cured in a moment that speaks of his alert consciousness, the more difficult one recovers, the weaker his consciousness is.

A lower than us animal, when it gets ill, it knows how to heal itself. And we, when we become ill, we call doctors, because we have no faith in God, nor in Nature, nor in ourselves.

One shall have a clear idea of the disease. Moreover, he should know how to treat it. For example, the stomach is treated by truth, chests are treated by wisdom and the head – by love.

At treatment, faith and will have to take an active part.

Tears heal – they clean the mind.

The duration of the Earth life of man depends on the relationships he has created by his soul. It is impossible for one to live solely for his personality and reach old age. The more the soul manifests its life, the more resilient human organism is. If one wants to recover, he must look for a doctor and medicines in his soul.

Occult Science provides various methods for treatment, for transforming negative energies into positive. Study these methods and make experiments with them to know which of them suit your organism. If you do not come upon the appropriate method for you, you may worsen your state. This is why some doctors do not let their colleagues treat them. I have heard a doctor saying: "I'm afraid to call a doctor, because he may give me a medicine that does not suit my organism and the state, in which I am. Here, I myself know what medications I have to take, but I cannot predict how they will affect my organism." So, any drug, even if determined for a specific disease, may has another effect on the organism. The best method for treatment is one to cope with his hardships and contradictions at every moment. One hardship may cause a certain disease. The contradiction may cause a certain disease, too. Therefore, eliminate hardships and contradictions from your mind in order to get also rid of the diseases, of which you suffer.

Gospel contains remedies for all diseases, all affected feelings, for disbelief and despair. However, you must know how to use these remedies.

If a person puts himself to a current of 2,000 volts, he will die, but if he puts himself to the effect of a current of more than 20,000 volts, he will renovate and clean himself without burning. Physicists say that the molecules of the current of 2000 volts are so great that by passing through the tissues of the human body, they destroy them and kill man. Molecules of the current of 20 to 50 thousand volts are quite small, as a result of which they pass freely through the tissues of the human body, massage them and instead of causing a trouble, they renovate and clean it. So, there are several types of warmth, light and electrical energy that affect differently the organisms. The smaller particles of these energies are, the more favorably they act - renovate, clean, and built the matter.

No pharmacy in the world can give people what Nature gives them. One must acquire magnetic energy from Nature and give from it to his fellows.

If one's stomach system is upset, it shall be treated by food. If his respiratory system is upset, it will be treated by light, warmth, electricity and magnetism. And finally, if the brain system is upset, he will be treated by thoughts and feelings. If you want to treat your brain, you should not allow inside any negative thought, grounding on the law that God is the absolute Love, the absolute harmony.

There are not only harmful microbes, but also such ones, which once introduced into the organism, improve it. In their practice, future doctors will use the benefits of those microbes.

While believing in the methods and drugs of ten doctors, the patient will never recover. To recover, he must believe only in one doctor, but healing powers hide in the water, air, light and food. Everyone is a conductor between Nature and himself, so he can heal himself alone.

When you heal yourself alone, you acquire confidence in yourself and your powers. If one leaves himself to a doctor, he relies completely on him and gradually he loses faith in his powers. Diseases are nothing, but tasks that must be properly solved. If they are not properly solved, then real diseases, which are healed with difficulty, come. Knowing that, do not be afraid of diseases.

If you want to heal one, who is ill, you should introduce into him the simple truth that he will recover. And by accepting that truth in himself as a seed, it will grow and give fruit. By sowing in you the thought that you are healthy, you will really be healthy.

Neurasthenia shows that through human nerves more electricity flows and that nervous system is shaken because of lots of work. In your bathrooms there is a faucet for cold water and one for hot water. If you open only the faucet for the hot water, you will be burnt. If you open only the faucet for the cold water, you will catch a cold. You shall open both faucets simultaneously and you shall carefully try until the water becomes pleasant for washing. Cold water comes from the head and warm water - from the sympathetic nervous system. You shall close a little bit the faucet of exceeding knowledge and open the faucet of Love. Knowledge and Love form a nice combination. If you have rheumatism – open the faucet of Love. If your shoulder hurts – pat it, become to love it.

Purity is one of the conditions for good health, for mind and feelings.

In order to heal someone, we shall free him from all alien elements, from all sediments that have deposited in him.

To recover, a patient shall clean his blood by breathing fresh air, exposing his back to the sun and by eating clean, healthy food.

You shall start from small microscopic experiments and gradually go to big ones, to great experiments. This method is observed also in science and in healing: from small to big results.

There is whammy in the world. For example, when somebody looks at you, you start feeling not quite well, you get a headache. There are people, who if they look at a bull or a cow, it immediately gets ill. The reason for that is the powerful look, which that person has directed toward you or to an animal, and that look is due to the electricity that comes out of the eyes of that person, which you cannot assimilate and that affects badly your organism. There are grandmothers, who know how to treat curses of the evil eye on people in the simplest way: they take one good egg and break it on the forehead of the bull or of the cursed person and he pulls himself together. Egg cures by absorbing the excess energy. However, only that grandmother, who is a good conductor of that electricity, may heal. Her organism shall withstand the impacts that come out of the ill person. The same may be said about doctors. Many doctors treat patients, but few of them have good results in healing. A true doctor must be a clue, through which the disease may get out. The doctor shall take and give something to the patient.

Any discomfort, either physical, or mental, is treated either by a method similar to the reason that has caused it, or by a method opposite to the reason. For example, frozen hands and feet are treated by coldness, and not by warmth. They are oiled with olive oil, because it absorbs the warmth in itself and thus relieves the body of the excessive energy that it has accepted by burning.

Create a harmonious environment for the patient and his spirit will calm down. One, who goes to an ill person, should not have any bad negative thought, because the patient is extremely sensitive; the doppelganger is extended and this produces one state of irritability. The doppelganger is extended with all neurasthenics. It takes a larger place than it is needed.

In order you to recover from a certain pain, stop talking about it.

Joy is life. In order one to recover from no matter what disease, he shall be joyful. He shall sing.

One may treat himself by connecting with healthy and good people, who love him. It is enough they to direct their thoughts and desires toward him.

I do not recommend patients to oil themselves with gas, I do not recommend drugs that peel skin.

As long as human eyes are fondled by hands, there cannot be happiness. Eyes are not made for being fondled by everybody. While eyes and heart are being fondled by human hands, there cannot be happiness. One may enjoy them from distance that they have a good master.

Neither give somebody to kiss your eyes, nor oil them with something. The only thing, with which you can oil eyes is pure water. There is water that is full of life-giving magnetism. It is clean, it refreshes.

One, who is ill, shall touch the lobe of his ear in order to recover soon and enhance vitality.

One should know that his body is a part of God's organism and if for preserving his life he ruins his brother's life, he depraves his life, too. What is the sense in cutting parts one after another and leaving only the corpse? Operations should be done, but not physically – the direction shall be from the physical to the mental. The method, used in modern medicine and surgery, is not correct. Before cutting a leg or an arm of the human body, first the reason, which causes the pain shall be found and eliminated. The reason shall be cut and the body shall be kept intact. Parts of the human body should not be cut.

To cut a leg of a man is not a science; to gouge out the eyes of somebody is not a science; to cut the kidney of someone is not a science. Some people say - a person may live with one kidney, but why Nature has put two? Doctors say that a man can live without a caecum. Nature has put it at its place, and doctors cut it, saying that one can live without it.

Surgery is an old science and cutting of the tonsils is an extreme method. The situation does not improve, but gets worse. What will fill the empty space? To restore something - that is science. To gouge the eye out, but to put a new one, to restore one's vision - this is surgery. Anyone can cut a leg, but to make a new one like the cut one – not everybody is capable of that.

Have patience to withstand surgery without anesthesia, because long time shall pass before one gets rid of the poison deposited by the anesthetic.

Cocaine is used during surgery and the patient does not feel pain, but the pain after the surgery is doubled. Nature does not like its energies to be suppressed. Do not think that you can save your sufferings.

You shall not sing to patients. When you go to someone, who is sick, you can pray for him, and he himself must sing. If the patient sings, you will sing with him; if he does not sing, you should not sing, either.

If you see that someone, who is ill, prays and sings silently to himself, you shall know that he will get better. The situation of a patient, who is not disposed to pray and sing, is awful. Such a patent will surely go to the other world. The disposition of somebody to a prayer and singing is a diagnosis, with which you can determine whether a person is healthy or sick, good or bad. When one loses that disposition, he roughens, becomes bad and soon he gets ill. Once softened, he begins to pray and sing. Not much time passes, and his health is restored.

If you have a headache, first put your feet in hot water, then clean your intestines.

I say that an ill person with high temperature shall keep a strict diet, eat nothing for 1-2-3-4-5-7 days. The room windows shall be wide open, more light to enter, and he not to sleep much; the mind shall be awake, to pray.

If you have a stomachache: you shall fast, eat less; every morning you shall drink a little cup of olive oil and one cup of hot water. Then you shall expose your abdomen to the sun, take the sun for 2-3 hours per day.

At cold, when you break into perspiration, you are out of danger. One has to sweat not only physically, but also spiritually. Sufferings are something like sweating. If one cannot sweat physically, he is in danger. And if he does not suffer, man is still at risk.

If you have fever or chill, you shall drink 1, 3, 4, 5, 6 cups of hot water or tea until you sweat well. Take off your shirt and wipe yourself; sit down and start again with several cups of water, oil your feet and hands with olive oil and go to bed. Another rule: take purgative to clean the stomach and intestines of all unnecessary substances, two days abstinence from eating, 3-4 cups of hot water, two cups of spinach juice with a bit of salt, two bowls of potato soup. You shall eat less.

If you have caught a cold, climb a mountain peak to sweat well, drink two or three cups of hot water and change your clothes. Climb peaks to induce deep breathing. This is especially good for those, who suffer from asthma, and those, who are prone to obesity.

When you cannot fall asleep easily, the reason for this is the excess energy in the brain. To get rid of it, you can do these exercises through which to send it to the other parts of the body: either by concentration of the thoughts to the tip of the nose for 5 minutes or through washing your feet with warm water in order to make some of your blood go down.

Why are there diseases in the world? They are educative. Through them the invisible world corrects people. If modern doctors were aware of that, they should teach their patients how to live. It is not enough just to touch the pulse of a patient and give him some medicine. No, hold the patient's hand and say: I will heal you if you are ready to correct your mistakes, to lead a clean life. And when the patient promises to correct his life, then the doctor will cure him. This is the way, in which doctors may do good to people.

Modern doctors study mainly the signs of diseases. Actually, a real doctor shall first of all know the signs and symptoms of a healthy organism to be able to compare them with the ill one. It is art to determine the diagnosis at least 10 years before a person gets ill in order he to take measures in advance. This can only be done by a doctor, who knows the occult sciences.

In my opinion, a real doctor is the one, who understands the reason for each disease and helps people. This is an assistant of Nature, who operates in accordance with its laws.

You should learn the language of organs. Each organ has its own special language. The liver has its own special language. The stomach has its own special language. The sympathetic nervous system has a special language. Muscles have a special language. Each organ has a special language, its own grammar. If you do not know how to speak in their language, they will not understand you. There are occultists, who use that language. Knowing the language of an organ, you can suggest it an idea. If your liver is upset, you can suggest it and after suggesting it, you will have results. You have become ill. You shall separate as a separate creature and talk to the ill organ. You shall say: "Do not worry, you will recover, you will recover, you will recover." You shall speak as if you are speaking to another person. If you say: "There it is!", you already suggest to the organ and your leg begins to hurt. You shall say: "You will recover. I will now put a bee, and when it stings you, you will surely get better." All people recover. When? When they become to believe. When a doctor treats an organ, he must know the language. If the doctor speaks to the liver, he can heal it. If he does not know the language of the liver, no medicine helps. One, who wants to be a doctor, he shall know the language of the relevant organ: liver, stomach, lungs, the nervous system.

What is the purpose of the doctor? It is to teach people those laws, which determine their health, their good life.

The purpose of doctors is not only in the ordinary way of healing. They have a higher purpose - to teach people to live properly, apply the laws of Rational Nature. In the future, doctors will be paid for each advice. Then they will not cure ill people, but they they will visit healthy people at least once or twice a week and will teach them how to live, how to improve their lives.

If you do not have love, the art of healing ill people fails. To treat ill people means to take off their backpacks from their shoulders. Sometimes it is better for one to get ill. If people were not ailing, they should come upon great misfortunes. Nobody can escape the suffering that Nature sends. If one avoids a suffering, he will be reached by two, three or more. Nature is rigorous and demanding.

If one goes to an ill person, let him first turn to God and say: "God, please, help me cure that ill person!" When one contacts the Divine consciousness, God already works through him. And when that person goes to someone sick, it is enough to put his hand on the head of the patient and after three minutes the patient will get out of his bed. That man already sees that there is a connection between him and God's consciousness.

When we go to treat an ill person and come into contact with him, don't we take some of his pain on ourselves? Do not think of that. At first you shall ask yourself: should I treat him? And if you have to treat him, you shall not yield to any consequences. How will we guess if we have to treat? If you love that person, you have to treat him.

It is not allowed everybody to be treated. If a spiritual doctor releases a criminal, he will bear his karma. There are criminals, murderers, who cannot be treated by a spiritual doctor by any method.

Christ never treated infidels or murderers and criminals. For such people there is no healing.

In ancient times an adept lived and he had the ability to cure various diseases. He healed deaf, blind and dumb people, who came to him. What was his astonishment when, instead of gratitude, they returned him cruelty and discontent. He turned to God with the words: "God, what is the reason, for which these people chase me? I opened their eyes and ears to see and hear, unlocked their mouths to speak and after all that I do not find peace because of them." God replied to him: "I closed their eyes, ears and mouths, because their hearts were cruel. To not sin any more, I deprived them of the benefits of the outside world. You interfered in my plan without permission, so, you will bear the consequences of this. It makes sense to open the eyes and ears of blind and deaf people, if they are willing to serve God."

The responsibility for treating for money is great. You will heal that person, take the money, but after one year he will die. And what happens then? He will instill in you and you will bear his karma. If you take money, you shall spend from yourself more than what you have received. Therefore, if you treat someone, you shall treat him for nothing. I tell you: the hand of the occult student should be pure, selfless.

One, who believes that he treats people by himself, he has the right to take money. But, one, who knows that God heals through him, he has no right to take money.

Food, light, air, and exchange with good people - this will be your medicine in the future. A good, holy person will treat you, without knowing that you are treated by staying with him. Doctors should be the best people.

If your stomach hurts, boil a little milfoil. Against cough - boil a little Gentiana cruciata and drink this water. If any of you has caught a cold, let him go up two or three times to a peak to sweat well. Then he shall drink two or three cups of hot water and change his clothes. Climb to peaks, to induce deep breathing. This is especially good for those, who suffer from asthma, and those, who are prone to obesity. The mountain hides within itself all the conditions for healing and learning.

Treatment by Food and Fast

Food is a method of treatment. There is not a better method than it, but you have to know what food to eat and when.

During illness and after the recovery one needs a specific food. For example, one, who has had fever, wants to eat sour food; one needs sweet food at another disease.

One thing shall be known: each Divine fruit has its great purpose. Therefore, if you eat apples, you will gain one quality; if you eat plums, you will gain another quality. One becomes what he eats.

Generally, oblong fruits represent intelligence, and knobby, round ones - life and feelings. Fruits are nothing else, but a combination of energies that operate in those forms.

Potatoes give only one quality to man – they make him happy and be satisfied by little. Apples give the following qualities to the human character: they make it soft, gentle, indulgent to people. One gains freshness. If you want to be sweet and gentle, eat grapes. In general, food affects one's character.

If you want to improve your blood circulation, eat cherries. What is there in cherries? Deep feelings are hidden there. The law of liberty is hidden in cherries.

What do cornels give? If you are spineless and slack and if you eat cornels, you gain stability and strength. They provide iron to the blood.

If the child is anemic, give him more pears; if he is a little bad, give him apples, if he lacks noble feelings, give him cherries, which simultaneously become a regulator of the stomach. Watermelons, cornels, and pumpkins also regulate the stomach. In general, fruits develop noble feelings. One shall just not overeat and overload his stomach.

Someone says: I have neurasthenia! Eat peas! Someone else says: I suffer from hypochondria. Eat wheat! They say for someone that he has a quick temper. Give him to eat corn! Someone is not persistent in the fulfillment of his duties. Give him to eat rye! There is something perfect in rye. It grows high up. When it comes in one, it develops supreme ideal.

Certain colors prevail in some fruits and in others they are less. For example, take the cherry – red prevails in it. And therefore, if someone is anemic and if he understands the law, while eating cherries, he will get, by no means, all that is necessary for his organism.

Apples originated in the astral world, and pears and lemons - in the mental one. If you look at the shape and color of a tomato, you will find out that it is behind in its development. It has not gone farther than the life of the stomach. Materialists are similar to tomatoes.

The cherry is a symbol in Nature. Red cherry, as well as all red fruits came out of Eden. Cherry is laxative to the organism.

For anemia - eat cucumbers.

One, who wants to be healthy, will eat not fried onion. Only one, who has chest disease, can eat fried onion as medicine. One, who wants to be healthy, shall eat food, cooked by someone, who loves him.

When onion is cut into small pieces and fried, it loses its magnetic power.

Cucumber has a beneficial effect on the nervous system, but it shall be eaten for breakfast and for lunch. If you eat cucumber in the evening, it affects the stomach badly. Generally, in the evening people shall eat before sunset. If one has not eaten by that time, it is better not to eat. Let him drink a cup of hot water or tea and go to bed with an empty stomach. In this way his sleep will be light and pleasant.

One, who wants to recover easily from cold in the head, let him apply the following means: when winter comes, let him buy at least 1,000 pieces of leeks and when he catches cold, let him eat leeks 3-4 times a day. Bulgarians are practical in nature, they look for remedies in folk medicine and they have come to the following results: if one catches cold in the head, he eats leeks.

If you have pain in tonsils, take hot garlic. This is a good way for treatment of tonsils and a good disinfection of the throat. Garlic influences excellently those, who suffer from insomnia.

Many people, especially Bulgarians, eat chilies. Chilies help against fever, but they are not recommended to healthy people. Too sour and sweet foods are not recommended either.

If you are nervous, indisposed, have two pears and two apples, small or large, the law acts alike. Power is not in size, but in the number "2" as a principle. Number two is magnetic. It mitigates energies.

You shall eat lentils for the eyes. For kidneys - beans. For nice tan of the skin - peas.

If you find yourself in physical discomfort, you should drink the juice of two or three lemons with sugar, and then - the juice of several oranges. The juice of lemons and oranges restores the good frame of mind, and improves the condition of the stomach.

Eat more spinach and nettles to darken your hair.

If your stomach is upset, boil cornels or eat them fresh. On the other side, cherries are laxative.

Everything that is forced brings bad consequences. You have read about the benefits of lemons and you treat yourselves by lemons. The lemon acid is healing, but you should know how to use it. Otherwise it causes cold, because it takes out the warmth of the organism, capillaries constrict, blood circulation is spoiled and one gets ill. One lemon per day is enough. Squeeze the lemon, fill up the cup with hot water and drink the juice. More than one lemon is not necessary.

It is not all the same whether you eat wheat, corn or oats. The energies of wheat are fundamentally different from the energies of the other cereals. One, who wants to become an idealist, shall eat oats. If you want to be healthy, obtain muscles, eat wheat. By the present, the most powerful and healthy food is wheat.

Sweet food gives softness to the character. Sour food gives activity and energy. Sour foods increase one's will.

One, who eats beans, will learn the law of generosity.

Cherries and peaches have healing properties. Cherries are recommended against anemia and neurasthenia. In spring, when there are cherries, you can eat as much as you like, but with love. In order to get benefits of the fruits, they shall be grown by a good person.

Each fruit has a healing power that must be used. If you are nervous, have three Petrovki apples (apples, which ripen around Saint Peter's Day

(June 29th) – transl. note) and the discomfort will disappear.

Apples are good for toning of the nervous system. Walnuts affect well the brain, and wheat has a good effect on the heart.

One, who wants to be happy and cheerful, let him eat cherries that ripen in early May. One, who wants to be a philosopher and wise, shall eat grapes – later fruits. When there are major difficulties, one shall eat turnip. It helps against many diseases. It is taken as a symbol of overcoming. When work does not go well, eat turnips.

Onion is healing when it is eaten raw, roasted or boiled, but not fried.

One, who suffers from neurasthenia, shall eat peas. One, who suffers from hypochondria, shall eat wheat; one, who is petulant, shall eat corn; one, who is unsustainable - rye. Rye develops high ideal. Small plants create people with small ideals, and large ones – the opposite. Villagers around Sofia shall eat rye to become greater idealists.

When one wants to disinfect his mouth or improve the condition of his stomach and his chest, he should eat garlic. I prescribe garlic to one, who is ill, but not to one, who is healthy.

If one wants to become a beautiful person, he should eat peas. If he eats beans, he will become healthy and will develop tenacity.

One, who wants to bring light thoughts to his mind, he shall eat fruits that have been grown in the north. One, who wants to bring nobility to his heart, he shall eat fruits that have been grown in the south. One, who wants to bring nobility to his character, he shall eat fruits that have been grown in the east. One, who wants to gain understanding for life, he must eat fruits that have been grown in the west.

If someone gets ill of arteriosclerosis, he shall eat, if possible, a little simpler and clean food. He shall eat boiled wheat, boiled rice and fruits.

When you are spiritually indisposed, make the following experiment: take half of a kilogram of fresh, big, nice cherries and go out at 10 a.m. before lunch. Turn to the Sun and start slowly and quietly to eat the cherries – for about half an hour; you shall eat nothing else, but the cherries.

For cough: you shall grate black turnip and drink one coffee-cup of its juice in the evening. It has an excellent effect on the stomach too. You shall also take a clove of garlic with a little bit of salt. You shall do this each evening until the coughing stops.

If the patient eats with gratitude and acknowledges that God cares for him, in the course of one month, his condition will improve.

People shorten their lives rather from overeating than from malnutrition. There are diseases that can be treated by hunger. But hunger is not always appropriate. Sometimes hunger has a good effect on healthy people too, but when it is as an internal impulse. Some people consciously put themselves to hunger, but they get scared and stop it. Then a certain poison appears in the organism. Know that you can survive with little food too. Hunger is an internal impulse with people, which makes them stronger and renovates them. If you hunger with fear and doubt, the effect is the opposite.

Fasting is for ill people, for sinful people, and not for healthy and righteous ones. Only one, who is ill, shall be treated by fasting. One, who is healthy, shall eat without overeating. Once he overeats, he has violated the laws of proper eating, because of that he shall fast.

The purpose of the fasting is thoughts and feelings of people to be filtered. On the other hand, fasting is needed for resting of the organism – external and internal rest. Fasting is also recommended as a means of healing. Within the period of fasting, burning in the organism is more intense, thanks to which all substances that cause various diseases, indispositions and dissatisfactions burn away.

If you do not get your language dirty by unclean words, it is fast. If you do not get your mind and your brain dirty by negative thoughts, it is fast. If you do not get your heart dirty by bad feelings and your will by bad deeds, it is fast.

One, who wants to purify his nervous system, shall fast at least four times a month. You shall know how, how long and when to fast. It is a whole science. If you purify your nervous system, you gain more light energy in your consciousness.

One is obliged to fast at least one day during the month, to give a rest to his stomach.

One, who fasts, shall not go for a walk. This is one of the rules. A student, who comes on a trip, shall carry bread, drink water and thank God. Everyone will be satisfied on a trip.

Leave a patient to hunger in order to wake up in him a desire for life. In this way he will recover sooner than if he eats.

Modern humans satisfy hunger through physical food. They can also eat air, but in a special way. How will they take in the air? Through the pores. However, the pores of modern people are clogged, due to which they cannot use the air as food. When their pores are open, the air enters through them and feeds the body. Then, by little food, they gain great power.

Fasting is used for renovation of the organism, for rejuvenating. After the fast, as longer as possible, consume unvaried foods and food, which requires little efforts for digestion, in order your appetite not to be stirred, in order lungs to be able to develop and take more food from the air and water, to take out more juices from food than now. The important thing is, through fasting, to achieve power, health, and not to show off and compete who can fast for more days. One, who has been fasting for 10 days, can do many things; one, who has been fasting for 20 days, will get rid of many delusions.

Fasting is a way of renovation of the human organism. The main idea of fasting is to awaken the hidden energy in cells and renovate the organism. But it shall be worked more rationally. Fasting shall be done step by step. There are certain laws that must be followed. If you make yourself fast, not knowing why, it is not useful. Time shall also be observed. Days, during which you will fast, shall be observed. If you start your fasting on Monday, you will have one result. If you start on Tuesday, you will have another result. If it is on Wednesday, Thursday, Friday, Saturday, Sunday - different results. Moreover, if you start fasting from the morning, from lunch time or from the evening, you again will have different results.

If you are not fulfilling God's will, nothing will be of benefit to you even if you fast for twenty days. But if you fast for ten days and each day you bring your meal, set for that day, to poor people, this fast can help you. Or, if you fast to eliminate one weakness of yours or gain good disposition of your soul, to purify your thoughts and feelings, I understand such a fasting.

With a 24-hours conscious fasting, one can renovate the cells of his organism.

If you decide to fast, you can begin the fasting when you are in an ascending degree of your spirit.

By fasting and a prayer you shall heal the diseases and weaknesses. However, if you are well-disposed, you shall fast longer, but if you feel exhausted, you shall stop fasting.

The stomach zone is related to the sympathetic nervous system. It shall not be loaded by excess alien substances. If this happens, you shall impose to yourselves fasting to restore the normal condition. Fasting should be moderate, reasonable until you remove the excess fats and sludge. Fasting means to abstain from bad thoughts and feelings - that fasting hides in itself magical power.

Hunger heals. If you suffer of rheumatism or another disease, you can recover by hunger. It shall be pleasant to you while hungering. Hunger detoxifies the body, pores open and breathing becomes deeper. Hunger brings more light to mind. Since ancient times people were treated by hunger.

You shall fast to restore your health, enhance the vibrations of your organism and your life.

Once a young man came to me and told me that he fell ill of an incurable disease. He was dying when he came upon a book for treatment through hunger and he began to hunger. He told me about the experience, which he had during the first day, the second and so on days until the 22nd day, and the result was that the disease disappeared. This person applied fasting for 22 days with faith in his mind and his heart.

I recommend to ill people at least 2-3 days of hunger, after which you can eat a little broth of plums (2-3 teaspoons), in a few hours - again, but with a little bread. When the patient gets stronger, I will give him a nice apple with the rind to chew it well with it to take all juices, and only after that he shall proceed to ordinary food.

All the misery is in your eating. If people knew how to hunger, they would have prospered.

If you are ill, you shall fast. It is necessary for you for a day, for two, and three. There are physical, mental, and spiritual fasts.

To get rid of his heartburn, one has to wash the stomach several times by warm water. If that does not help, let him fast for two or three days. Fasting cleans the stomach, relieves it from excess heartburn.

When a wound occurs in the organism, it is well one to put himself to an absolute fasting for several days.

Fasting is a method, by which a person solves great and difficult tasks. You shall fast not one, but 40 days, during which time, you shall clean your mind, heart and will – you shall not leave anything unclean in yourself. Someone has fasted for 10 days and thinks that he has done something. He has not eaten roasted chicken and has not drunk wine – what kind of fasting is that? When you start the fasting, you shall take the old notebook and eliminate something each day. You shall forgive all people. You shall fast and pray.

By fasting one strengthens his will and gets rid of the fear that he will die of hunger. Hunger heals. Rheumatism is treated by hunger. Hunger detoxifies the body, pores open, breathing becomes deeper, the light of the mind increases.

It is good from time to time to eat only raw wheat. I will give you the following experience: those of you, who have weak stomachs or bad chests, let them put themselves to a wheat diet for one, two or three months at most. During that time no other food shall be eaten, nor bread. Only well cleaned and washed raw wheat shall be chewed. This experience shall be applied only by those, who are nervous and indisposed and want to be treated. If you think that one month is too much, make the experiment for a week. You shall soak in the evening 100 g clean wheat in water and divide it into three equal parts: you shall chew in the morning, at noon and in the evening; if you get thirsty during the day, you can drink as much as you want. If you had put yourselves to that diet earlier, you would have had healthier teeth and your nervous system would have been better regulated. If you feel something disharmonious while doing the experiment, stop it.

Treatment by Water

If you understood the properties of water, you would be able to treat all diseases by it. Water, by which you will treat yourself, must be absolutely clean.

A big part of the human body is water. Many people suffer with lack of water in the body. Moisture, water is the reason for the warmth of the body. The lack of water cools the body. Too much water heats it. One has to live properly, use reasonably the energies, coming from the Sun for creating a healthy and pleasant atmosphere round people. If one lives well, he attracts to himself the flows that come from the Sun and forms an oasis - a source of life and powers.

If you want any drugs, either as remedies, or means of cleaning, I would recommend the following: drink each day 2-3 liters of clean hot water. If you are up and about, carry water by yourself. Carrying of water is beneficial to the organism. Furthermore, take deep breaths to expand your lungs.

Hot water, taken in sips, cleans the nervous system from deposits, which clog thoughts and feelings of people. It releases them from the tension that the nervous system establishes in them.

I say: the most powerful medicine in the world is hot water. And if we know where the best springs are, we shall bring it from there, even if they are at a distance of 5-10 km. Modern people do not know what power there is in water.

Modern people do not know how to drink water and how much. Each organism needs a certain amount of water that shall be contained in the cell to maintain its moisture. If the organism loses its moisture, it is exposed to drying. Such people are usually nervous, dry, and irritable. Without the internal moisture and the outside water, one cannot clean his organism from the external and internal deposits. If these deposits remain in the organism, they will cause undesirable diseases. If you want to be healthy, keep in your mind the thought of the beneficial effect of water on the organism. Drink water consciously and do not think about diseases. Keep in your mind the thought of your health, of the beauty and great things in life and do not be afraid of anything.

Nature has put billions of windows in the human organism – the pores, through which the vital energy penetrates and constantly renovates it. These windows should always be clean and open in order proper exchange between the internal and external air to happen. If the windows become dirty, if they get clogged by various deposits, the organism is already exposed to diseases. The pores of the body are opened by water, which causes sweating. Magic power hides in water - it cleans the body, dissolves sludge, and is a good conductor of magnetism.

At certain diseases, massaging of the whole body is recommended till sweating. Sweating is caused by a reasonable power, which wants to show you that all pores of the body should be open. The first treatment, which needs sweating, washing of the body. Perspiration happens in the best way by drinking of hot water, boiling water, from 1 to 10 cups at most. At drinking hot water, it goes through the pores out, opens them and this restores health. Pores are channels, openings of the soul. Soul breathes through the pores. Through lungs a specific breathing is performed, and through the skin pores, general breathing happens. And when the specific and general breathing happen simultaneously, one is healthy.

Water is highly intelligent and reasonable. It freshens and refreshes. Future physiologists will explain one of the great properties of water, by which people can be treated. Many neurotics suffer with lack of water in the organism, with very little moisture; others suffer with stagnant water, which does not spread throughout the body, because it is clogged.

You will take the glass of water, will look at it, and get it close to your lips and take only one sip. While drinking, you will think only about it. Water cleans the organism only in this way. It introduces the Divine good in people only in this way. You will take water internally for cleaning. Modern people do external water baths, but the result is weak. If one does not make regularly, three times a day – in the morning, at noon, and in the evening – by one internal bath with clean water, he may not rely on any hygiene. In the way you perceive water, in the same way you will perceive light and air. It means to be healthy, well-disposed, and satisfied.

Due to unnatural life, people have accumulated in their organisms lactic and uric acids, which are harmful to the heart and circulation. Then one will fidget for hours in bed, he will not be able to fall asleep. How could he sleep in this situation? For sleeping well, he needs to improve his circulation. For this purpose, at least twice a week, one shall induce sweating by drinking water: one shall drink several glasses of hot water, in which a few drops of lemon could be squeezed. When he gets well perspired, he shall wipe the body by a damp towel and change the clothes. He shall sweat again, wipe again by a dry towel and so on until sweat stops coming out. After that let him drink another half or one glass of hot water. It helps for releasing the blood from the accumulated in it lactic and uric acids. To be a healthy person, one shall have absolutely clean blood.

There is no a better medicine in the world than warm water, but you should know how to boil it. The most reliable medicine is warm water. Quinine is nothing compared to water. You shall get clean spring water, put it on quick fire, in a vessel of the purest gold, and boil it at sunrise or when the Sun is at its zenith. Other medicines only clog the disease. The most powerful drug in the world is hot water. People should know that water is the first element of life, and shall always drink clean and fresh water. Life is hidden in water. And when it disappears from your body, it dries, as well as the skin. Sour by nature people have less water in their bodies, and phlegmatic ones have stagnant water in their bodies. Water in the organism must be in current state.

Quinine stops the fever, but does not heal. Instead of using quinine, drink hot water for three days without eating and the fever will leave you. Cold in the head is treated in the same way.

Water heals all weaknesses in the world. Watch the effect that water has on the organism of someone, who is irritated and indisposed. In what way? By drinking of hot water or by washing the body.

Plague is treated by hot water. One, who is ill of plague, shall be separated from healthy people and be given, every hour, a glass of hot water. While drinking the water, the blood serum, which serves as food for microbes, thins out, and they gradually stop multiplying. During the disease no food should be eaten. The relationship of man with God is a power that affects microbes as electric lightnings. Thus, attacked from both sides by firing and hunger, they stop multiplying and die. A 24-hours hard war against microbes of plague is enough to compel them to come out of the organism. Diseases are nothing, but a war of man with lower beings.

I treat cholera by hot water. Give one, who is ill of cholera, 4-5 cups of boiling water and on the next day he will be healthy. Boiling water thins out the serum, in which germs of cholera eat and within 24 hours they decrease and die.

Influenza comes to take away the excess ballast from the human minds and hearts; when it comes, drink hot water, eat boiled potatoes and do not be afraid.

If you have a headache, drink three cups of hot water in sips. After that you shall take a purgative. When you liberate your stomach, you shall take a warm bath and go to bed. You shall stay a little in the bathroom. If you have a headache, your stomach also suffers by all means. Sometimes one suffers from his head also because of insufficient blood in the head – in the brain. Indeed, the there should not be much blood in the head, nor less, but as much as it is necessary.

When blood vessels in somebody lose their plasticity, their agility, he gets ill of atherosclerosis. One, who wants to keep his health, to prolong his life, he must keep his body mobility. For this purpose, one should not overeat and drink hot water, which helps sludge, which form during eating, to be dissolved.

If someone suffers with stomachache, let him make the following experiment: in the morning he shall drink 10 sips of hot water at every five minutes; if he does it several times the stomachache will disappear.

If you have a constipated stomach, take castor oil or drink hot water to get rid of the difficulty.

If you are indisposed, take a warm bath. Water influences magnetically the organism.

If you catch a cold, put hot compresses on the ill place. Dip a piece of cotton in boiling water and quickly place it on the ill place for 1-2 minutes. Then put it again in the boiling water and from there on the ill place. After making this compress for about ten times, the pain will pass.

It is good partial baths to be made. Sometimes they are even preferable to entire baths. Louis Kuhne recommends to weak and ill people sitting baths: only half of the body to be washed and the other half to remain dry. If one day you wash yourself to the waist, the next day you will wash from the waist downwards, or if you wash your face in the morning, at noon you will wet your head slightly at the back. In this way proper exchange in the body is caused. Proper washing of the feet will affect the arms and vice versa. Furthermore, while washing your feet and hands, do not be in hurry to wash them as soon as possible. Rapid washing shows misunderstanding of the law. Dip your feet in the water and sit for a while in this position. Mentally wash your feet until you feel some pleasantness, a reaction in your hands. Then slowly wash your feet. By washing in this way, the powers of the organism distribute properly. Some people take a warm bath and then go to a cold shower. These abrupt changes on the body are not for an average person. They are only for gods. One, who is not hardy, shall take only warm baths, leaving the energies of warmth affect his organism. Cold showers that occur in Nature are good, but only under certain conditions, and namely the rain baths in May, June, July till the middle of August at most. If you cannot take rain baths, take warm water baths of 34-40 degrees, close to the natural warmth of the body. It is good rain baths not to be made straight on the body, but through a thin article of clothing. Do not wash your feet by cold water by no means, especially after meals.

If the amount of salt in the human body is more than it is needed, the excess shall be thrown out. It happens through sweating.

Water bears life, but it is not the same with salt. Eat little salt.

Nature does not tolerate cold showers, cold baths. Warm baths are preferable to cold ones.

Some people recommend cold compresses, and other – warm ones. When cold compresses are put on the ill place, capillaries contract, as a result of which specific reactions in the organism are induced. If warm compresses are put on the ill place, the responses are beneficial. Warm water causes blood vessels to dilate, resulting in improved blood circulation.

When someone is extremely agitated and nervous, he can take a cold shower. Water releases people from excess energies in their organisms. For an angry person, the water temperature must be above ten degrees. In order he to cope with his anger, he shall take at least six cold showers during the year. In this way, he will balance the powers of his organism. One, who is angry, loses part of his energy, which is hardly delivered. Reasonable people keep their energies and do not spend it randomly. One, who gets easily angry, ages faster.

If you have cold in the head, warm a little water, put salt in it, and sniff up several times from the salt water. You need to do some more sniffing-ups in the evening and in the next morning. After 2-3 snuffs, the cold in the head passes. Salt water hampers the multiplying of microbes that cause cold in the head.

If you cannot fall asleep for a long time, wipe your body by a towel dipped in warm water and go to bed.

You should know that the rain in the mountains in July is a great blessing. Such a rain bath is equivalent to one hundred ordinary baths. Every drop of rain in July is full of electricity and magnetism.

From May until the middle of July, each day when it rains, you will expose to the rain until you get wet well. After that you will return home and wipe your body by a clean towel, get dressed in dry clothes, and drink 1-2 cups of hot water.

Dew is to be collected in little bottles and sealed by wax. It shall be collected for treatment. Early in the morning, on absolutely clear days, when the Moon is getting full in May and June

How drunkenness can be treated? Make the drunkard drink 2-3 liters of water a day and he will recover. In the process of healing, he should start with the least quantity of water and increase it gradually: the first day he shall drink a glass of water, the second day - 2 glasses, the third day – 3 glasses, then 4, 5, 6 glasses until he reaches 15-20 glasses a day. If he fulfills these instructions, soon he will abandon alcoholic drinks. When the drunkard comes to love water, he will stop drinking wine and brandy.

Washing is a sacred act. Wash yourselves slowly, intently – you will take a clean basin, pour cool water, rinse your face well, absorb the moisture very slightly by a soft towel. You will splash your face abundantly with water, but gently, affectionately, as though you pet it.

Face is gentle and responsive and therefore you will barely touch it. After washing, you will look at yourself in a mirror and if you are not happy with the face, wash it again.

Before and after the end of each work, you shall wash your hands, and you shall wash your face at least ten times a day.

Water, with which you have washed your face, shall be thrown to the flowers, the trees, but, by no means, at a place, where people pass or at unclean places.

When you go to a clean spring, you will wash your hands and feet away from it, you will sprinkle your head, drink some water, but you have no right to throw stones in it or other objects. This also applies to rivers, lakes, wells.

Washing of the various parts of the body produces psychic changes in the brain. You can not only literally use water for treatment, but even if you mentally use it, it will produce the same effect. For example, you want to make a water bath of the spine, you will imagine a fountain at a distance from you, and you will get there, fill the pitcher with water, come back, take off your clothes and wash your back.

You will wipe the moisture by a soft towel.

Treatment by Breathing

The air is a store of Divine energies. Air is the largest store, in which life has stored its energies.

I say: the air bears Divine thoughts that first pass through the respiratory system, where they are processed, transformed and from there, by blood, they go to the brain. So, one cannot perceive the Divine thoughts directly through the brain. Air is the main bearer of thoughts. If, in the current conditions of life, air is taken away, one could not perceive any thought. In this sense, breathing is sacred. Therefore, one has to breathe properly in order to be able to perceive the Divine thoughts from the air and deliver them to the brain after that.

Each Divine energy, which comes down, must first pass through the respiratory system and go up to the mind from there and then down to the heart.

Breathing is different with every person. It is determined by the degree of his development. Patients usually breathe faster. Animals also breathe faster. A healthy person breathes smoothly, quietly, depending on his development.

No matter with what disease you suffer, look for help in deep breathing. There is no disease that cannot be treated by breathing. Long life depends on the deep and proper breathing. On the other hand, breathing depends on the right thinking and feeling. Breathe deeply and think that God's blessing comes on people through the air.

Breathing is a dual process: physiological and psychological. The ultimate goal of breathing, also as mental process, is cleaning of mind.

The lung is a complex laboratory, in which lots of energies cross. Prana from the air enters the lungs and helps for the ozonizing of blood, even where it is hard for the air to penetrate. In the so cleaned blood, elements of life are introduced.

Since the air is saturated with light and prana, while breathing, one accepts these two elements necessary for blood.

Besides through the stomach, a person eats also through the lungs and through the brain. Through the lungs and brain he gains energy from more sublime food than the physical one. A day will come when people will eat only through the lungs and through the brain.

When someone gets ill, his breathing becomes faster. It is easily noticed mainly with people with thin chests. When their breathing becomes difficult, they consciously accelerate it, thinking that this will help them. They do not help themselves, and their condition even worsens. This shows that in order one's breathing to be normal, it shall correspond to the natural rhythm in Nature. This rhythm is healthy.

Proper breathing depends on the quantity of the taken air and the time, for which it is kept. The longer someone keeps the air in his lungs, the more powerful he is. On this depends also the success of his undertakings. Some adepts have come to the point to keep the air in their lungs for half an hour or even for one hour.

People, who have lost their balance, breathe very fast.

At faster breathing, the oxidation of blood is quicker, so part of it cannot be cleaned and that is why many people have more venous, unclean blood. At quicker oxidation of blood, the burning in the organism is improper, as a result of which some of the combustibles cannot burn away and accumulate in the form of sludge along the arteries and veins.

Man has seven million pores, through which he connects to the air, and in addition, the lungs, which are directly related to the air.

If one does not breathe properly, the skin of his face and hands prematurely get wrinkled. Wrinkling is due to a disorder of the liver and improper breathing.

Concentration of the mind depends on breathing. The deeper one breathes, the easier he concentrates.

There are special breathing techniques for every person. One may reach to these techniques by his internal teacher and doctor. Listen to your internal doctor, i.e. to the Divine in you.

Now, by talking about deep breathing, I do not intend recommending specific exercises. Hindus have special breathing exercises, which are not applicable to Europeans. That is why I say to you: breathe deeply, aiming to breathe smoothly and rhythmically.

One thing should be known. Many of the Hindu rules and methods do not meet the ones of the living, reasonable Nature. For example, if in the West the science of breathing, which is applied by the Hindus, is applied, it will give negative results. Why? It is because these systems are acquired in the course of descent of humanity, i.e. after the law of evolution. And since the white race began its development after law of involution, i.e. in the way of ascending, these systems need to be modified.

Hindus work hard on deep and full breathing. At that lots of energy is collected, which Europeans do not know how to use. Finally, instead of good, they will bring something bad to themselves.

The Scriptures say: "And God breathed into his nostrils the breath of life and man became a living soul." Hence, he breathed in air through the nose and accepted the Divine life. Therefore, when one finds himself in difficulty, he must breathe. The air is a bearer of electricity and magnetism. This energy passes through the nose and renovates the nervous system. By breathing you can make the brain think properly and the stomach operate normally. Improper breathing is the cause of many diseases. Leg hurts, because you do not breathe properly. The same concerns the head and the heart, as well as the spine. The fast and shallow breathing is dangerous - leads to various diseases.

The vital power, prana, which is in the air, cures. There is a power between love and life – this is prana. Prana renovates the mind. When you breathe, think that you take in prana through all cells. When you breathe, you will not think about your wife, your children, and anything that is not connected to breathing. You will leave aside the cattle, bees, eating, this one or that one. By concentration of the mind, you can recover from any disease. By concentrating your mind, you can protect yourself from a bad fortune that comes to you. The bad fortune moves like a projectile and you can move at only three or four fingers aside of its way and the projectile will pass without touching you.

The more one keeps the air in his lungs, the more energy he obtains from it. By breathing in this way, the unclean air will not affect him badly either, because he takes in less air and therefore less dust and dirt. When the number of breaths decreases, life prolongs, and vice versa. If you get to one breath per minute (in and out), you have acquired a lot. Breathe with joy and love, with a smiling face, straight; your spine shall form a parallel line with the line that joins the center of the Sun to the center of the Earth. Your chest - forward, thrown out, and not hollow inside. By breathing properly, you connect with the rhythm of Nature and strengthen your spirit and your body.

In the lungs there are plant cells that need carbonic acid and therefore, through deep breathing, by holding the carbonic acid in the lungs, these plant cells strengthen and prolong their lives. By holding the carbonic acid for longer in the lungs, one strengthens the plant cells in himself. And if he strengthens them, he is healthy.

Health is associated with conscious breathing. Therefore, at least 3 times a day (in the morning, at noon and in the evening, before going to bed) one must spend 10-15 minutes to breathe. By breathing, he must thank for the air, which he takes in, as well as for the good that is in the air. This means conscious breathing.

Breathe deeply to take as many of the life-giving prana. Prana has different conditions: physical, cardiac and brain, or mental. Without prana, thoughts cannot be formed. Without prana feelings cannot manifest and finally, without prana will cannot function. Everyone, depending on his development, will take what he needs, and will express what he is able to.

When one breathes, he has to appreciate air as an invaluable good. First love affects the lungs. One, who loves, expands, and his lungs expand too.

Now, when I am talking to you about the proper pulse, about the rhythmic beating of the heart, the question about the proper deep breathing pops up right away. Almost all people breathe improperly. They breathe in and out only in the upper lungs. At this shallow and weak taking in of air, they have no power to take it out, as a result of which part of the unclean air remains in the lungs, where internal accumulation happens. If one wants to regulate his blood circulation, he has to breathe deeply, hold it for a while in his lungs and then slowly take it out. At breathing, the abdominal muscles shall also take part, give a push, tension to the air and take it out. By breathing properly, one renovates himself and gets rid of both physical and psychic painful states.

There is a prana that is absorbed through the left nostril, and another one that is absorbed through the right one. Through the left one the magnetic flow is taken in. It is connected with the solar plexus and is called a solar flow. Through the right nostril the electrical flow is taken in. It is connected to the cerebrum and is called a lunar flow. If we want to develop the mind more, we take in air through the right nostril and take it out through the left one. And when we want to develop the heart more, we breathe in by the left nostril and breathe out through the right one. When we change the way of breathing now through the left nostril, now through the right one, we balance both flows, as well as the electricity and magnetism.

So, breathe deeply, consciously. If you do not feel well, if you are sad, breathe deeply. If your spine hurts or if your waist hurts, breathe deeply. If your leg hurts or if your arm hurts, breathe deeply. If you have a headache or a stomachache, breathe deeply again.

When one does not take in enough prana from the air, he feels weak, exhausted, without energy. Who is guilty for that? He alone is. It depends on him to take in more prana, because it exists in Nature abundantly.

By living on the Earth, one needs air as food for his etheric doppelganger, for his astral body. The air contains a special energy, called prana by the Hindus. Other scientists call it life-giving electricity or life-giving magnetism. You have come to the mountains not only for clean air, as many of you think, but you have also come for prana. You go out early in the morning for taking in the particular light rays of the Sun for prana of the mind and its heat rays for prana of the heart. Lungs take in prana from the air best in the morning.

It is noticed that the deeper one breathes and the more he holds the air in his lungs, the wider his nose is. Flattened nose indicates that one's breathing and circulation are weak. If the nose is very sharp, one is nervous, irascible, and irritable. To calm down, he should breathe deeply.

One is afraid of breathing in cold air to prevent against colds. If the air is taken through the mouth, you are right to be afraid. However, Nature has foreseen that, too. It has made nose to serve as a filter for the air and warm it. The mucous membrane and fluid in the nose regulate the air and make it bearable to human lungs. In addition, when you go out when it is cold, do not rush to take in much air at once. You will take in air little by little until you adjust to the outside temperature. You will breathe bit by bit, you will take in little air and gradually increase the amount of air. In proper breathing there is a certain rhythm that must be followed.

While breathing, you will breathe in slowly, calmly, without haste. When you take in a certain amount of air, you will hold it in your lungs while you are taking in from it that vitality, which it hides in itself. There is no greater blessing for one than slowly breathing and holding of the air in the lungs, while taking in the vital power, i.e. prana, which it bears.

Ordinary breathing should reach 15 breathings in and out per minute. By doing the exercises, you will aim to gradually reach one breathing in, one holding and one breathing out per minute. If you achieve that, you can cure all diseases, even tuberculosis. Do the following exercise: hands clenched into a fist, put on your shoulders. Slowly open your arms to both sides, breathe in deeply, hold the air and then let the arms go slowly down along your body and slowly breathe out. In this way you take in enough prana from the air and the blood gets going, the capillaries dilate and circulation increases.

As disciples you should treat yourselves by deep breathing. If you have a stomachache, do six exercises four times a day. When you do the exercises, put your left hand on your stomach with the palm down. Put your right hand on your left hand, palm down again. By breathing in deeply, you shall feel the shrinking and relaxing of the diaphragm. One, who does not breathe deeply, cannot be a disciple of the new doctrine.

Breathe easily, smoothly, with a certain rhythm. Make attempts to treat yourselves by breathing in the morning, before lunch and before dinner by 12-19 exercises. Each breathing in, retention and breathing out is an exercise. By doing these exercises, your mind should be concentrated, the diaphragm shall go up and down, shrink and relax. The diaphragm is a boundary between the spiritual and physical worlds. One of the causes of palpitations, shortness of breath and some chest diseases is due to the displacement of the diaphragm from its natural position. If it is raised higher than it should be, the heart and lungs do not operate properly. When a person takes in a deep breath, the lungs are filled, press the diaphragm and it takes the defined for it place. You can breathe and read "Our Father" or "The Good Prayer". You will breathe slowly, deeply, without deviation of the mind. One, who is not exercised in deep breathing, let him keep the air for two or three seconds and gradually increase each day the retention by one more second until he reaches 30 seconds. If he can keep the air for 30 seconds, he will cope with many indispositions and diseases - headache, chest disease, stomachache, paralysis - everything disappears. Treat yourselves before you have become ill. If one does not breathe deeply, no medicines can help him. One, who breathes properly, his breath and sweat smell nice and the circulation is normal. No matter with what disease you suffer, look for help in deep breathing. There is no a disease that cannot be treated by breathing.

At breathing, the abdominal muscles shall also take part, give a push, tension to the air and take it out. By breathing properly, one renovates himself and gets rid of both physical and psychic painful states. It is good to breathe in by the left nostril first, by counting from 10-15, then close it and keep the air in your lungs for about 30-40 seconds and then breathe out and rhythmically. When you breathe in through the left nostril, the right must be closed, and while keeping the air, both nostrils shall be closed. These exercises are necessary for all people, especially for those, who deal with mental work. They are necessary for both healthy and ill people.

Breathing exercise: arms are to be opened slowly aside while deeply breathing in, then they are to be raised up, keeping the air. Arms behind the head, slow put them down while breathing out slowly.

Breathing exercise: Slowly raise your arms above your head and breathe in deeply. With the raising of hands, eyes are also lifted up. Hold the air for a while. Slowly put the arms down, breathing out and slowly take the eyes down.

A breathing exercise. Both arms spread aside, horizontally, with open palms facing up.

1. Inhaling - slowly breathe in air while bending fingers, at which the thumb is to be put over the middle finger and over the forefinger. During that time you are thinking that along with air you are taking in also the love of God. It penetrates into the air and everything, because God penetrates in everything, and God is love.

2. Holding of the air - as long as it is possible, while thinking that we assimilate love; it penetrates in our entire nature. During the retention of the air, slowly get your arms back with bent fingers and put them on your chest.

3. Exhaling - slowly stretch your arms aside, horizontally and when they are completely stretched, slowly unbend the fingers. Meanwhile breathe out and think that you send light that comes out of our love in the world.

A breathing exercise. Breathing in - 16 time units, holding of the breath - 16 time units, and breathing out - 32. You will do this three times a day – in the morning, at noon and in the evening by 6 repetitions. You will breathe in through the left nostril, hold the air, and breathe out through the right nostril. You will do this for 2-3 months.

A breathing exercise, the aim of which is to increase your ability for holding air. You will not use any time units at this exercise. You will breathe in slower and deeper, and then you will hold the air as long as possible, and will breathe out as slowly as you can. The retention time is to be gradually increased: 1 min, 1 1/2 minutes, 2 minutes, 2 1/2 minutes, etc.

When you are nervous or angry, do the following exercise: close by the thumb of your right hand the right nostril and breathe in through the left one while silently counting to 7. After that do not take in any more air and silently count to 10. Then close the left nostril and slowly breathe out through the right nostril, counting to 9.

This exercise helps for regulating the nervous excitement, for calming the brain and strengthening of the memory. In the morning and before lunch breathe in through the left nostril and breathe out through the right one. In the evening breathe in through the right nostril, and breathe out through the left one. You will do exercises by 21 times a day: in the morning, before lunch and in the evening by 7 repetitions.

Breathing exercises of another nature. In these exercises there are certain thoughts, certain formulas, which have to be silently said. For example: while breathing in, holding the breath, and breathing out, you can say the following words: "Thank You, God, for the blessings that you have given me." You can silently say: "Our Father" while breathing in, as well as while holding the air and breathing out. You can do such exercises in the morning, at noon and in the evening by 10 repetitions. You can also silently say: "The Good Prayer" - 1 time in total. You can silently say while breathing in the words: "power", "life", "health" (3 times). You will do the same while holding the breath and while breathing out. You can do this exercise in the morning, at noon and in the evening by 10 repetitions.

When you take in the air, you will silently say the word "life", while holding the air, you will pronounce the word "power" and while you are breathing out, you will think on the word "health". You will slowly, calmly breathe in, hold, and breathe out again slowly, while you are thinking on the above words.

Living energy, which is to refresh our organism, comes through the spine. The spinal cord has the quality to absorb prana from the air and transmit it to the whole organism. Write down the formulas that you can silently pronounce while breathing in, holding, and breathing out:

Breathing in: "Thank You, God, for the Divine life, which You have introduced in the air and which I take in together with the air."

Retention: "This Divine life that I take in with the air penetrates in all my cells and spreads power, life and health everywhere."

Breathing out: "This Divine life strengthens me and I show this out through my activity." Under Divine life it is understood prana. You will vividly imagine how prana oozes from cell to cell, from organ to organ and spreads everywhere.

Breathing in: "Let God's name be glorified in me."

Retention: "Let the kingdom of God and His righteousness establish in me."

Breathing out: "Let God's will be done."

Breathing in: "Thank You, God, for coming in me."

Retention: "Thank You, God, for being in me."

Breathing out: "Thank You, God, for leaving your blessing in me."

Breathing exercise. You will breathe in through the left nostril. At that time the right one will be closed. While breathing in, you will silently pronounce the formula: "Only the love of God is love." By holding the air for a while, you will open the right nostril and slowly breathe out by saying the same formula. At that time the left nostril will be closed. Do the exercise three times a day: in the morning, at noon and in the evening when you have time. At each exercise you will breathe in and out 3 or 10 times.

Exercise. Breathing in through the left nostril. During this time the words: "Let God's name be glorified in me." are silently pronounced. While holding the breath, the words: "Let the kingdom of God and His righteousness establish in me." are pronounced. While breathing out, it is pronounced: "Let God's will be done." It shall be breathed in through the left nostril 5 times. Then the opposite - 5 times it shall be breathed in through the right nostril and breathed out through the left one.

Treatment by the Sun

The energy of our physical, mental, and even moral life comes from the Sun. It brings life.

Only the solar energy is able to restore one's strength and health.

There is no disease that cannot be treated by the Sun.

The Sun's rays are a collection of billiards of rational beings, who come to an expedition to the Earth. Each rational being leaves his signature on the faces of people. They call these signatures tanning.

The Sun is a source of living energy for the whole solar system. With respect to the Earth, the solar energy is positive. It develops in positive and negative electricity and in positive and negative magnetism. The Earth energy is negative with respect to the Sun. The Earth has both energies, but mostly negative. The Sun also has both energies, but mostly positive. As a result of the contact of these two energies the life on the Earth was created. The mediator that unites and transforms these energies is called ether. It penetrates into the space and the entire Earth. The occultists call it life-giving plasma. The mystics call it spirit.

The Sun contains all the drugs in itself. There is no disease that does not submit itself to the effect of the sunbeams.

To heal, one has to pass the sunbeams through certain prisms. These prisms can be physical, but they also can be mental.

The solar energy descends on the Earth as a vast stream, encircles it from the North Pole to the South one and goes back again to the Sun. This energy is transmitted to plants through life-giving plasma. When plants become to feel that this potential energy begins to manifest and come to the Earth, they bud, prepare, and when it increases, they put forth leaves and finally blossom and knit, while trying to gather all that energy to fecundate themselves.

Wise man, seeing that his body is lacking some energy, collects it from the Sun. He knows that the Sun can provide any deficiency of energy in the human organism.

Energies, which the Earth accepts from the Sun, transform significantly. By penetrating in the Earth layers, the latter absorb from them all nutrient elements and only what cannot be used remains. Transformed in this way, these energies are not useful for the development and therefore they are sent from the Earth into the cosmic space and go back from there to the Sun along certain paths. The Sun sends them to the Central Sun for further processing in order they to obtain their initial rhythm. From midnight to noon Earth is negative (actually a certain place) and that is why it perceives more, and from noon to midnight it is positive and therefore it gives more. From midnight Earth begins to radiate in the cosmic space negative energy, and, at its place, it accepts positive one from the Sun. At sunset, Earth is the most positive and therefore it gives most. In the afternoon it starts to radiate into the cosmic space positive energies and when it has radiated enough quantity, it becomes negative. In the morning, at sunrise, the Earth is most negative, i.e. it perceives most.

We are a part of the Earth organism and hence, when it accepts, the human organism also accepts. Therefore, the first beams are the most effective ones. Then the human organism is most receptive to the solar energies. In the morning, we always have more prana or vital energy than at noon. Then the living organism perceives most and most powerful positive energies. The first sunbeams are the most active ones. This life-giving high tide is the strongest till noon, then the low tide starts and the strongest one is at sunset. An hour before sunrise, the energy of the Sun has a psychological effect on the cells of the body – it renews their energy and creates new impulse for work in them. Before sunrise the beams, which are refracted by the atmosphere, have a greater influence on the brain. During the sunrise, the sunbeams, coming in a straight line, have an impact on the respiratory system and our sensibility. The same beams affect the digestive system. Hence, the healing effect of the solar energy is different: before sunrise – improvement of the brain nervous system, at sunrise – for strengthening of the respiratory system, and from 9 to 12 o'clock - for the stomach. In general, in the afternoon, the solar energy has small healing results. The reason for this difference is the different perceptive ability of the Earth and of the human organism.

The energy that the Earth takes from the Sun can be compared to the arterial blood, and the one, which it sends to it, can be compared to the venous blood. Our Sun plays the role of a heart and that role is better played by the Central Sun. In the way, in which the unclean blood from the tissues has to go back to the heart and from there to the lungs for being purified, the energies of the Earth return in the same to the Sun to acquire their initial rhythm.

The solar energy passes every day through 4 periods: from 12 midnight to 12 noon, there is a high tide of solar energy, and from 12 noon i midnight there is a low tide. The high tide comes to its highest point at sunrise. This high tide is the most powerful and life-giving.

To meet the rising of the Sun is to consciously connect with it, in order its powers to be able to flow through your body. If one connects to the Sun of the physical world, he connects to two more suns at the same time – the Sun of the spiritual world and the Sun of the Divine world. If one does not meet the rise of the physical sun, he cannot be healthy. This law is known not only for people, but for all living beings.

The reason, because of which our Sun burns us is the following: a black zone of the evaporations of our thoughts, feelings and desires forms round our Earth and those burning sunbeams form as a result from that. Therefore, we perceive the sunbeams through reflection.

By studying the influence of light, you will notice that there are hours during the day, when the Sun sends to the Earth beneficial beams, mainly in the morning until noon. There are hours during the day when the sunbeams are not beneficial to the organism. These are the so called black negative beams. In order not to fall under their influence, beware not to sleep during the day. The disciple should not sleep during the day, especially when the black sunbeams are active. If he sleeps during the day, he feels unwell, tired, depressed. One can expose himself to the sunbeams during the whole day, but his mind must be focused, positive, to perceive only the positive sunbeams. You will concentrate, but beware of falling asleep. Along with the black negative waves of the Sun, Earth waves come, too and they influence badly one's organism. Until you learn the rules of fencing, keep away from those waves. It is best for you to sunbathe within the early hours of the day, not later than noon. Beware of the afternoon sunbeams. When you want to treat yourself by the sunbeams, the best hours are from 8 to 10 a.m.

Christ recommends the Sun as a method for treatment. When the day is not sunny, you will cure in your room – you will bandage the wound with olive oil and onion, and when the Sun is shining, you will go out, untie your wound and expose it to the Sun.

If the exchange between the energies of the Sun and the energy of your body is proper, you will always be healthy. Only one, who is healthy, can understand the ideas of the new doctrine.

God put the Sun in the sky, which to shine on you, and you look for your doctor to artificially heat you by a lamp. This is not healing. If you sun yourself every day, consciously, for half an hour, with the participation of the mind, you will get more than if you rummage through books for days looking for what doctors say about a disease.

Wise man, seeing that his body is lacking some energy, collects it from the Sun. He knows that the Sun can provide any deficiency of energy in the human organism. When a certain organ, either leg, or arm paralyzes, or the sight fails, or the memory fades, this is due to not sufficient energy, not enough income of blood, food to that organ. Wise and rational man would not say: "God's will is such.", but will get right away what is needed, will gather energy, and will heal himself.

If one does not get tanned by the Sun, this indicates that he is not healthy. The Sun cannot heal him. Proper exchange shall happen between the Sun and people. The tan shows that the Sun has taken out from the human body the whole sludge, dirt, and dense matter. If one does not tan, that dense matter remains in the body and causes lots of diseases.

If you tan by the Sun, this means that you have accumulated its energies. Tanning is a sign that you have taken energies from the Sun.

If a person does not have gold in his blood, the Sun cannot heal him.

The more gold you have in your blood, the more you can have outside of yourself. The amount of the external gold is proportional to the one in the blood. If there is gold in the blood, the organism is healthy, the mind is fresh and sober, and the feelings are noble. Gold is a stored solar energy that Hindus call prana. Prana is necessary. Health depends on it. That is why it is recommended one to go out early in the morning when he can take in more prana. Ten minutes are enough for a person to stay out at dawn and sunrise to take in what he needs.

Furtively you will cast a glance at the Sun for one-tenth of the second.

The Sun acts too strongly and in order not to damage your eyes, do not look directly and for a long time at the Sun. The light is not bad, the retina is not adapted.

If you had knowledge, you could perceive from the Sun so much energy to heal every disease. If you knew how to use solar energy properly, you would have made by now the grains of wheat as large as eggs and if you knew how to use properly the solar energy introduced into the grains of wheat, you would do everything! You have to study the energies that come from the Sun.

If at the rising of the Sun you understand that you perceive more of God's love and more of the Divine life, then the sunlight will be healing for you. If you do not think and realize that thing in this way, the sunrise will be for you purely a mechanical process that will not be of benefit to you.

Our organism is made of billions of cells that, on the Earth, they have the property to perceive the sunbeams, transform them and retain from them the needed for renovation and healing prana. If you do not feel well, go out, expose your back to the Sun and you will get from it what no one philosophical thought can give you.

When you sunbathe, it is well if you are dressed in white or light green clothes - these colors are nice. Perspiration is the important thing. If you are at an open place, cover yourself by a thin mackintosh. If you treat in this way, you should focus your mind to heal directly from Nature.

Mountain sunbathing is preferable, because the rhythm of the Sun is not disturbed by the astral mental cloud that covers the city.

The Sun does not function in the same way during all seasons. The Earth in early spring is more negative and that is why it receives more. So, in spring, sunbeams are the most healing. From March 22nd onwards, the Earth gradually becomes positive. In summer, it is already too positive and that is why it receives less. The summer beams influence too, but less.

The best months for renovation are from 22nd March, throughout the entire April and May till 22nd June. Any growing stops on the latter date.

There are days in the month of September, which with reference to the vital energy, are equal to the days in May. Use the sunbeams during these days. Then light beings present around you.

Many illnesses are treated by the solar energy. Moreover, it is proven that for every disease there is a certain time when it is treated. Some diseases are treated in May, others - in June, July, generally, during the whole year.

The sunbeams in the morning from 8 to 9 a.m. are the most healing ones. At noon the beams are too strong and do not have a good effect on the human organism. Early sunbeams influence well anemic people.

When one wants to use properly the sunbeams, he shall expose his back under a certain angle. If this angle changes, he will not benefit of the rational sunbeams. Speaking of the Sun, we do not have in mind only the physical sun, but also the spiritual sun as a manifestation of intelligent, rational powers, as a manifestation of beings - bearers of love and wisdom.

In future, when people understand that, they will be treated only by sunbeams. They will know which beams against what kind of diseases and weaknesses can be used.

Under the influence of the Sun cosmic consciousness in man awakens.

The energies that come out from the Sun hide in themselves a reserve of vital powers, of healing energies. If one wants to use wisely the energies of the Sun, he has to expose his back to the early sunbeams, before the rising of the Sun. Energies that he will take in at the time, are equal to the energies that he would take in, if he exposes during the whole day to the Sun. Even on a cloudy day, you can go out before the rising of the Sun and concentrate your mind in the direction of the rising Sun. Clouds only prevent you from seeing the Sun, but its vital energies pass through them. No external force is capable of counteracting the energies of the Sun.

If you have an eczema, if your hair falls, if you have rheumatism in the joints or any swelling in the abdomen, if you are rich, built a terrace exposed to the Sun and surrounded by windows, take off your shirt to the waist, lie down with your head to the north and feet to the south, expose your chest to the Sun, keeping your head away and remain in that position for half an hour. Then the back – half an hour, then again the chest - half an hour and continue in this way until you get well sweat. If you make 20-30-40 bathes, everything will disappear. You can expose to the Sun your entire body. You shall sunbathe in the morning from 8 to 10 a.m. If these bathes have an effect on the spine, brain, lungs, you will feel the effect on the whole body. The brain is like a battery. When that battery begins to take in, if the filling up with solar energy happens properly, after that it sends it to all parts of the body and that energy begins to heal.

The more solar energy you take in yourself, the greater softness and magnetism will develop in you.

When one puts his hands with palms facing the Sun, this can warm the entire body, because the warmth of nerves passes throughout the entire body.

Go out under the Sun every morning, exposing your back first to the south, then a little to the north, a little to the east and stay in that position for one hour from 7 to 8 a.m. Direct your mind to God and say: "God, enlighten my mind. Give health to all people, as well as to me along with them." Then start to think about the most beautiful things you know. Do this experiment during the entire year. You will see that 99% of your experiment will be successful.

The good effect of the Sun on humans improves the state of the arterial blood. The Sun raises human thoughts and feelings, thanks to which human blood cleans too.

There are such diseases, which do not submit to any drug, but disappear once you expose them to the quiet sunbeams. Lumps, bumps will disappear after 2-3 months. When one connects to God, when the Divine light comes, the lumps gradually disappear.

I say that the only best surgeon I know is the Nature - the sunbeams. Only they cut most appropriately – they cut the rotten meat most properly without affecting the healthy one.

When you want to treat yourself, expose your back to the early sunbeams. When you want to gain internal peace of mind, expose your back to the going down Sun and face eastward.

I have often said that one should communicate with the light. If your back hurts, expose it to the Sun, to the light, think about it, about what it contains and the pain will disappear. All diseases of the mind result from deficiency of light, of the heart - of deficiency of warmth. All diseases of the soul result from deficiency of truth.

When one gets ill, he has to connect with the energy of the Sun and the Moon. If he cannot contact them directly, let him use the plants and minerals that are associated with the energy of the Sun and the Moon and transform them properly.

Do not look at the Sun when it shines strongly. Watch it in the morning when it rises. There is also a particular way of taking in the sunlight, not only through the eyes. Few people can use properly the light, air and water. Most people breathe only by their lungs. There is another way of breathing - through the astral body or through the etheric doppelganger.

Whatever discomfort you have, if you expose your back to the Sun, the discomfort will disappear. If your discomfort is due to negative thoughts, expose your back to the south and the face to the north. It will not take long before your discomfort disappears. If you have caught a cold, expose your back to the south, to the sunbeams. They heal all diseases. If the energies, which have produced your discomfort, are positive, turn your face to the south and your back to the north and the discomfort will disappear.

Treatment by Colors

Each disease is treated by light - red, blue, yellow, orange, violet. The light is selected in accordance with the disease.

It is not important for you to live in the colors, but in the energies of those colors. One, who wants to transform his life, he must connect to the light itself, to benefit from its energies.

The most beautiful colors can be found in plants. Plants are the greatest art exhibition. They are pages of the great Divine Book.

The external light that we see is a result of the mind activity of the higher beings, who are above us. It comes out of the eyes of these beings. Animals perceive the light, which comes out of us.

The effect of the colors depends on their vibrations. The higher the vibrations of a color are, the better the result is. When you do not feel well, you should know from where this indisposition comes, in which color you are and by which color you can help yourself.

Light manifests by vibrations, but the vibrations themselves are not the light. Thought also manifests through the brain, but the brain does not create the thought.

Humans know only seven colors of light, without being aware of the fact that they are to know 5 more colors. Humans may see only 12 colors of light on Earth.

The more yellow rays there are in the brain, the better one thinks. When the thought is not awake in him, he is deprived of the yellow rays. The first three rays of the seven ones have an impact on the physical life; the second three rays affect the spiritual life. (Under 'spiritual life' it is understood the ability of someone to realize things inside himself as they manifest in the physical life.)

Even before getting ill, one can be healed by the colorful rays. The seven colors represent seven sacred worlds that send by one colorful ray. The seven colors are the solar spectrum. The more intense the color is, the closer the world that sends this color is to us. From the rainbow colors we can guess toward which area we move. Which color is dominant on the Earth? It is the green one. All creatures on Earth are immersed in green. At the same time, we are connected to all planets and suns, as well as to the beings that inhabit them.

Each color has its own purpose, which learned people know. For example, the green color is materialistic, the red is active (it is mainly an animal color), the orange is a color of the extreme individualism. The only colors that correspond to the current development of people are the light blue and the light green ones.

The red color, on its part, is composed of seven colors with different intensity of vibration and different number of vibrations. A person with a well-developed eye may distinguish seven nuances of red and benefit of them reasonably. These nuances are negative and should be turned into positive. They represent a written book that should be unriddled. One, who can distinguish the seven nuances of the red from each other and benefit of each of them in accordance with the relevant qualities, he will feel completely refreshed.

You are ill. Your illness is due to deficiency of light in your organism. How will you recover? By accepting the needed light in yourself. Each disease is treated by light - red, blue, yellow, orange, violet – light is selected in accordance with the disease. No matter if you suffer with deficiency or excess of light in your organism, you are exposed to irregular conditions - physical and mental.

The seven nuances exist in the different worlds in different octaves and differ in their influence and importance. They mean one thing in the physical world, and another in the other worlds. At its low manifestation, the red light means a struggle, an element. All creatures that, in one way or another, have stored in their blood that light, are extremely active and rude. Cold is a small amount of light. Behind the ordinary light, other energies of higher type stand, and behind the latter something rational stands. The clean red color produces life, vitality, cheerfulness. The clean orange color gives noble personalized service to God, and the unclean one - doubt, disbelief.

The clean yellow color gives balance of feelings, peace, serenity, intellect, and in its low manifestations - use, self-interest, everything for personal purposes, foxiness. The clean green color - growth in every aspect, and in its low manifestation – drying, attachment to the material. The light blue color – boom, extension of feelings, most sublime feelings, and faith. In unclean form – doubt, disbelief, vanity. The clean dark blue color gives calmness, firmness, decisiveness, and in its unclean nuance - inconsistency. The violet color, the clean one, gives power, used for higher purposes, fortitude, and in unclean form – power, but used for personal benefits.

Light speaks to people simultaneously in seven different languages. Each color of the light has a specific language. One, who understands these languages, is healthy, learned, strong or if he is ill, ignorant, weak, through these rays of light, he can recover, because each color is associated with a certain type of powers of the human organism. Thus the red color is associated with the powers of the heart, the orange one – with the powers of the mind, and the green one – with the powers of will, the yellow one – with the powers of the soul, the blue one – with the powers of the entire sky, the violet one – with the powers of the spirit.

Many people suffer with intoxicants: wine, brandy, tobacco, and others. There are intoxicants in mental life, too - some thoughts and feelings intoxicate like alcohol. One, who does not know them, takes them in and gets ill after that, suffers until he gets rid of them. Sometimes the reason of diseases is the lack of a certain color in somebody. If he lacks the red color of love, the yellow color of wisdom, or the blue color of truth, he will certainly be ailing. They can be introduced both in the organism and in the psyche.

The more intelligent one is, the clearer his light is. If intelligence is reduced, the light becomes slightly bluish, then pale yellow, etc. The level of human intelligence may be guessed by the color. When you come to the heart, where love is, you will see there a particularly tender nuance of the pink. At the same time, it also emits pleasant mild warmth. Finally, when you come to the will, white color of virtue comes out of people – the color of virtues. Between these three colors (light, white and pink), the rest colors intertwine. This intertwining of colors is the human aura. Through the aura, the clairvoyant guesses how far a person has reached in his spiritual and mental development.

Red affects the human aura, makes him active. Orange affects one's personal life, makes him an extreme individualist. Yellow gives space and peace of mind.

The more you go into the dark colors (e.g. in the dark blue), the more sadness and grief are felt in the soul. The effect of the light colors (light blue, light yellow) are soothing to the nervous system. The blue color is a medium for the spiritual life of people. The green color regulates the magnetic and electrical flows in the human organism. It is related to growing. One, who wants to grow, to be healthy, he must get connected to the green color. The violet color is related to the will of people.

Here is what I will recommend you for healing and rejuvenation: buy a prism, about half a meter long and 20 cm wide, put it in your room and focus your attention on one of the colors in accordance with the disease you have. If you have anemia, you will choose the red light of the spectrum. You will pour over with this color about ten days. If your stomach is upset, you will select the green rays of the light. If the nervous system is upset, you will take the light blue rays. The colors of the light may heal all diseases.

Work with the colors, with the various nuances as methods for treating and gaining of those energies that are missing in your organism. All people do not need the same type of energies, so not everybody like one and the same color. If you do not have objects to connect you with the various colors, work mentally, by saying such words, which will awaken in you the relevant colors. For example, if you say the word "blue", you imagine right away either dark blue, or light blue. The first one is a color of the valley, so it gets you low in the valley of life. The light blue color reminds you about a sky, height, so your thought is raised high to a mountain peak. The rest colors also produce different states of the human thought.

One, who has developed extreme sensitivity or suffer with neurasthenia, let him use the blue color of the light. Every morning pour with blue rays of the light over your head, chest and stomach.

Generally, it is well one to direct blue, yellow or orange rays to those organs of the body, in which he feels an excess energy. Sometimes, at some places in the human body, a certain blockage appears, which creates abnormal conditions. You shall pour over your body with the blue and yellow rays of the light. Humans may accept these rays from the Sun. Initially, you will use a glass prism. Through this prism you can get the solar spectrum on a wall. After obtaining the spectrum, you shall focus on the blue color and try to take it inside yourself. Then close your eyes and see if the same color can imprint in your mind. By doing these exercises, you may, whenever you want, produce blue, yellow or another color in your brain and treat yourself. When doing these experiments, initially great darkness will establish in your mind. After a while, in your brain as on a screen, a little light will flare up as the dawning on the horizon. This light will gradually increase until it strengthens so that it can heal.

Cleanness is the best cure for all diseases. The basic tone of life is obtained through cleanness. Red cannot be obtained without cleanness. Cleanness is a bearer of the red color. Red bears that material, of which life is built. The red color, which you see, is only a shadow of the real one. The red color of the rainbow is not the basic red color. The red color will bring in you joy, warmth, light and power. Once you perceive it, you immediately feel that you have gained something.

If you bring the red color in the organism of someone, who is anemic, the red corpuscles in his blood will start to increase and life in him will strengthen. If you bring the orange color in the human organism, he becomes independent, begins to think freely. If the green is introduced – one starts to build, to create. In every color, Nature has hidden certain types of powers and the reasonable person, knowing that, can obtain what he lacks through each color. By taking in the red color of the light, one can obtain a healthy and beautiful face. There is no a better cosmetic effect on the human body than the red color. There is no easier, more natural way for improvement of the health of people and gaining of vitality than the taking in of the red color. Lipsticks, powders, and pomades clog pores, atrophy and spoil cells. If a child blisters, powder may be used, but there is no need of powder on the face of a healthy person. The face must be beautiful, plastic.

Until the taking in of the red color, one will be exposed to a number of painful states. If you do not take in correctly the orange color, you will lose your individualism. If you do not take in correctly the green color, you will stop your growing. If you do not take in correctly the yellow color, you will stop your mental development. If you do not take in correctly the blue color, you will begin to degenerate in religious aspect. If you do not take in correctly the violet color, you will gradually start losing your will.

The white color establishes health in man. The white color brings health. Black evokes bad, negative conditions in man. When one is ill, he has to dress in white clothes. One must constantly change the colors. Colors evoke movement, life. They are energies, which have different effects on people. One has to go through all nuances of the range of colors. Furthermore, it is defined how much time he shall spend in each color, in each nuance of the range of colors. If he spends more time than the defined one in a given color, certain satiety will settle in him.

Black is a color of relaxation and concentration: after working all day, one needs to rest for a while, collect his thoughts, and give nothing out. It is not a bad color. Psychologically its effect is nice. It is a color that collects more energy. When a person is very nervous, it is better for him to wear black clothes to have more energy. Children are dressed in white. It is correct and appropriate, because they have plenty of energy to distribute.

If the heart is ailing, harmonize with the red rays of the light, take the red color in yourself. If the thoughts are disharmonious, the yellow color has to penetrate in you. If the liver is upset, you shall take in the green color. All colors may be separated very well by a prism. A reasonable power in Nature stands behind each color.

If a person has more of the red light and the other lights are missing, then he has a predisposition to anger.

When you suffer with headaches, eye problems, rheumatism, or any other disease, do experiments with the colorful rays to see how they will affect your organism. There are many ways, in which you can treat yourself, but treatment by colorful rays is amongst the most effective ones.

When you want to heal a certain weakness in yourself, pass the pink and yellow colors through your mind.

Light colors (light blue, light yellow) are soothing to the nervous system. Green regulates the electric and magnetic flows in Nature and in the human organism.

Fear is a negative quality of the lower mind and if it heavily occurs with someone, it is better for a person to take in the orange color as a means of balancing of powers. He can recover through it.

You are discouraged. You are in a deadlock. You are not able to think. Use the yellow color. Select the yellow color of the light and do it so that it to shine forth in your mind.

No one of the colors shall be watched for a long time.

Blue brings calmness in man; sky-blue has an especially smoothing effect to the nervous system.

One, who has little faith, let him introduce the blue nuance in himself and remove the disbelief. Power goes through the violet nuance. You will use pink, when you do not feel well, and for health - red.

It is well to take seven silk threads in a notebook, which to correspond to the seven colors of the spectrum, and look at it at any indisposition. Nature treats by colors.

I say: what you know about the application of colors with regard to clothes of the people, concerns also their thoughts and feelings. Each thought, each feeling, each action is dressed in a certain color like in an article of clothing.

Treatment by Music

Music, in the physical world, is needed for organizing the disorganized matter. The physical world is disorganized. Through music matter vibrates harmoniously.

Music is a Divine way for success in the world. Through music higher beings reach us. You, if you sing, will contribute for more advanced creatures to come and help you. If you do not sing, they will not be interested in you.

Occult science recommends singing as a method for converting the negative energies into positive.

Music organizes the body and from there - the thought. It organizes the thought and from there - all cells. Music raises the vibrations of the organism.

Music is used from long ago as a method for transforming of the energies and for treatment.

Singing is an appeal of the human soul to Nature. Being responsive, it sends its reasonable building powers toward a person to help him recover sooner.

Today music can be harnessed as a method of treatment. If you make somebody, who is ill, sing a little every day, he will soon recover. On the other hand, if one, who is healthy, stops singing, he will easily fall ill. Music is the boundary between the physical and spiritual worlds. Through it, man can transform his energies. Through a song, a particular vital energy flows into the human body. If you are nervous, indisposed, start singing. Your condition will change right away. By singing such abilities are developed, which may not develop in another way.

In order one to be healthy and develop normally, he should gain an inner balance between the powers of the matter, of which his body is made, as well as between his thoughts and feelings. Music is one of the means for maintaining that balance. One, who knows the laws of natural music, can stop the destructive activity of the parasites in his body and improve his condition.

Singing is not entertainment, it is a means of toning up the energies. You shall sing to gain certain energies. If a patient does not sing, he will die prematurely. He should sing to provide the lost energy to his organism.

When one sings, he has to put in the song his soul and his spirit. They change the vibrations, raise them, and each increase of the vibrations has a healthy effect on the organism.

When you sing, Love, Wisdom and Truth must take part in your singing to express everything that God has put in you.

Many of the modern doctors, particularly in the West, treat patients by music. Bulgarians are pessimist by nature, that is why they have created horo-songs to take treatments for their pessimism. Joyful music has a healthy effect. There are sad songs that may make even a healthy person ill. Bulgarian horo-songs are healing.

At each pain capillaries contract. When you start singing, expansion happens and that contraction of capillaries stops, pains stop.

Music is a way for transforming human conditions. There are conditions that cannot be changed without music.

You have not used music yet as a means for healing and developing of your abilities. Through music you can produce power in yourself, remove discouragement, or remove your pains. You will sing one, two, three, four, five times a tone or the entire scale and you will see how your situation will improve. Someone has robbed you. There is no need of telling here and there what has happened to you or searching for the thief. You'd better say to yourself: "Wait, I will give a concert."

Musical tones are related to the human organism. The brain has its own specific tones and vibrations. The heart has its own specific tones and vibrations; the stomach has its own specific tones and vibrations; the liver has its own specific tones and vibrations; the muscles and bones of people also have their own specific tones and vibrations. In the future, music will play a major role in healing.

One, who is ill, has to sing during the whole day to recover, and one, who is healthy shall also sings to keep his health. The more correctly a person sings the tone "re", the more the condition of his lungs improves.

Heart represents the tone "do", the respiratory system – "re", the liver – "mi", the kidneys – "fa", the spleen – "sol", the gall – "la", the digestive system – "si". When the respiratory system of somebody operates musically in all scales, we say that it is normally developed. At the least violation of this system, its tone changes, goes to another tone, and this creates disharmony in some of its organs. This disharmony is called disease.

Once the vibrations of the stomach decrease, a stomach disease comes. Once the vibrations of the lungs decrease, lung disease comes. Then you can use music to raise the vibrations of the body and recover.

There is music, which tames beasts. There are songs, by which you can treat yourself and by which you can expel death. Death fears and flees from those songs.

One, who sings, gets ill less. If he gets ill, he easily recovers. In this sense, music is a good remedy.

Sometimes I go to a patient and I look at him while he is alone and I see him singing for while, then he cries for a while, but his cry is again in the form of a song. I know that this crying is music and say to myself: this person will recover. If he stops singing, he will not recover.

If a patient sings to his illness, he will recover. Without music and singing, one gets demagnetized. Soul is also toned by music.

You often complain of illnesses and sufferings. I say: sing to diseases and sufferings. If you are ill and you cannot move your arms and legs, sing. Noon comes - sing. Sing to your illness during the entire year to see what the outcome will be.

One, who knows to sing properly, he can heal himself and his fellows. The different diseases: headache, chestache, rheumatism, etc. are healed by different music.

The material world comes from chaos, and that is why it is disorganized. The solar world organizes the unorganized matter. Rheumatism is unorganized matter, accumulated in the joints and impeding the circulation. You will sing to that matter. By singing, a movement is created that clears mud. Singing is a powerful flow that cleans the entire organism, but only that singing, in which every cell, every fiber sings, Nature sings, birds in May sing, the fragrance of flowers is singing.

Once you get ill, do not be afraid, do not seek outside help immediately, but begin to converse with the disease. Ask it from where it has come and what it wants from you. When you understand its intentions, sing for a while, do not chase it, it will be your guest for while and it will go away. Everyone wants to be healthy, but does not know how to gain health.

There are patients, who are treated by playing a violin, others – by playing a guitar, third ones – by playing a flute, etc. The various instruments have a specific impact on each person. If the patient likes to listen to a violin, you will play to him for a while, but with ascending vibrations, and not minor songs.

Tachycardia is treated by songs that start with the tone "do", not the one taken by a pitchfork, but the natural tone "do". If you take that tone correctly, you will immediately feel calmness in you, little joy as if you have gained something. No matter how little that joy is, it brings into your soul light, shining as if the Sun has risen. The basic tone "do" is the key to life. Everyone can do experiments in that direction, to verify that truth. When one wants to sing, first he must adjust himself to come upon the natural tone, the natural key. He will stand upright, remain calm for 10-15 minutes until he gets rid of all difficulties and contradictions that exist in his mind, will ponder over the reasonableness of life and then start singing. This means that this person is able to turn properly one of the musical keys given to him. That also means the sun to rise in him and the reasonable energy to start flowing in his organism. If the tone "do" is properly taken, one can take the life-giving energy in from the Sun and transmit it to all organs in his body.

If you have anemia, take frequently the tone "do". It is a tone of life. You will introduce a little gold in your organism through it.

One, who is a little stubborn, rough by nature, shall play Chopin. He will deliver mildness to him. One, who has lost the meaning of life, shall play

Bach. One, who does not want to read and does not like to think, shall play Beethoven. One, who does not like poetry, shall play Mozart. Each musician is a good fruit and you will choose one or another according to your frame of mind. It is not one and the same whether you will eat apples, pears, cherries, grapes or another fruit.

The words "zum-mezum", in occult music, regulate. They are resultant forces that regulate everything. So when you want to tone yourself, you may sing the exercise "Power alive, spring, flowing".

At home, make a patient sing and he will recover. Make him sing "Sweetly, honeyed", then the other exercises. He can recover in this way.

While cooking, you shall sing. While digging a vineyard, you shall sing. While sowing and reaping the field, you shall sing. Singing is a formula. Singing is the right thought.

If you are ill, if you are hungry, sing the song "Goodness, goodness".

After each disturbance, a disease comes. When two people quarrel, cold or a wound, or infection comes. In that case, sing "Sweetly, honeyed". However, not all diseases can be treated by music.

If you are ill and poor, if you cannot see a doctor, and do not have money, sing a song like our song: "Life of our soul, which fills up the entire Earth, is beautiful". Sing it three times and you will recover. Then sing "In the beginning was the Word". Is it real that I will recover once I sing it? Will you recover if you do not sing it? Sing it, do not hesitate. If you sing, you will recover.

In the future, doctors will treat by music and songs. You laugh at that, but people are unaware of how ridiculous and distorted they are without music. Music in relationships, in movements, in feelings, in thoughts, in deeds.

Treatment by Mind

Diseases may be treated by thoughts. The mind may expel any disease from the human body.

Words are powerful. So is the human mind. It is enough for somebody to apply consciously, with faith, his thoughts to experience that power. Will is needed for that. Through thoughts people, suffering with incurable, horrible diseases, are healed. As long as one believes in the power of the mind, he can do wonders with it. However, strong will is needed for that, without any hesitation.

If people knew the laws that govern the human mind, they could cope with all weaknesses of theirs. There is no a weakness, which could not be fixed by the mind.

Not only the beings from other planets and civilizations influence the Earth, but all people, who are about three billion, affect the Earth and Nature by their brains. The brains of all people affect the entire structure of the Earth. If people concentrated their minds on a certain point, they could melt everything that is there. Rock would be melted by the energy radiated by the human brains. People, if they knew how, could melt all sorrows and diseases by concentration of the mind.

The organism has certain vibrations when it is healthy. The vibrations of the various diseases are different. However, each disease means that the vibrations are decreased. The temperature should be increased. This happens by special thoughts and formulas that change the vibrations when one introduces them into his organism. This is achieved by looking at beautiful paintings and landscapes. The night sky may also serve as a remedy. One, who is frustrated and sick, shall look at the vibrating with different lights stars. One may encourage and recover through the starlight.

Each word has a certain power. If you focus your attention on a word, your brain will connect to the power that is in it and you will experience encouragement or fatigue depending on the nature of the word. There are words that once spoken, cannot be pronounced again. Why? They have a harmful effect on the human brain. For example, if you pronounce several times the words: "I will get ill.", you will experience their bad effect on your body and it will not be long before you may get ill. And conversely, if a tubercular patient repeats several times a day the words: "I will recover", he really will.

People may treat themselves by the mind. The stronger and focused the human mind is, the easier one may recover from a disease. It is enough for him to say a word to recover. There are words that have a magical effect on humans. You shall also know when to say the word. Everything should happen at its place and time.

Diseases are due to accumulation of alien substances, but, by the mind and will, people may throw them out of the body and recover. The more sublime a thought is, the more opportunities it hides in itself.

According to the occult science, every word has its own specific key. If the key of the word "health" is found and if somebody, who is ill, pronounces it 3 times, he will surely recover. By pronouncing the words correctly, you will discover the power contained in them.

Strong mind heals all diseases. Kabbalists explain treatment through thoughts in the following way: thoughts are able to modify the vibrations of the human body. When a person becomes ill, these vibrations lower; through thoughts people could turn them from lower to higher ones. The cold in the head is caused by a particular type of microbes, which get into the nose, and if the vibrations are lowered, they find conditions for reproduction. When their number increases, they begin to irritate the mucous membrane of the nose, and the nasal glands, in order to get rid of this irritation, produce plenty of fluid, which throws them out. Once the vibrations of the body increase, the throwing out of the alien substances is easy and fast. By the mind, one may intensify the cold, to lead it to the utmost limit of its development, after which it begins to decrease. The longest period is one week. It should not remain more than that time.

The matter of the physical world submits to the human will. For this purpose, you need to know the laws that govern the will. The matter submits also to the human mind. Therefore, apply the energies of your will and thoughts. Through the efforts of the will and thoughts, one may take the alien substances out from his body. While these substances are in him, he feels physically and mentally unwell. Once he applies his mind and begins work consciously, soon he may make the alien matter go out from his organism as a furuncle. The furuncle is burst and the impure matter flows out.

As disciples, you have to work with your minds, to do experiments, to use the hidden powers in your organisms as remedies. There are cells in people, the task of which is to heal. They are called healing cells. It is enough for somebody to direct his mind to them in order they to show their effect. Only a concentrated and positive mind is needed. Every negative thought paralyzes the function of the cells. If one wants to recover, he shall maintain positive thoughts.

I say: a disciple shall concentrate, develop his mind, but not in the way of the yogis. There are many ways and methods, which yogis use, but if he does not understand them, he may totally cripple himself. These crippled disciples are beyond the laws of Nature. The laws of rational Nature are severe. I give methods that are associated with the least risks to the human mind. They are the methods of the living, rational Nature. The yoga methods, however, are associated with great risks.

Concentration happens with open eyes. You will heal yourself with open eyes. You will think of your hands, your feet. You will pass your mind through the nervous system, the stomach, the intestines, through the entire body as a master, who shall go for a walk all over his property to see in what situation everything is. This is concentration.

When a Hindu concentrates, he does not think about his wife, his children, his bees, about anything else, but prana. A Bulgarian thinks about the cattle, the sheep, his wife, and his children; about this and that, due to which he has no good results. He is unable to concentrate. However, by concentrating the mind, you may recover. You may divert a misfortune, which comes against you as a shell. You may divert the beast that prowls you.

The human mind is related to the vital electricity in life. When the thoughts are positive, they attract the vital powers. When the thoughts are negative, these vital powers disperse and go away from you, as a result of which a disease appears. For example, if you have an enemy, who hates you, his thought of you is very strong. He may make you negative and you will become ill.

The law is the following: if you get ill, that disease will go back to him. There will be a reversal.

You can send your positive thoughts, your warm feelings and wishes for a patient with an absolute faith, without any hesitation and doubt and he will get better. So, in order one to be healthy, you shall send from yourself a vital current toward him. He will take in your thoughts and wishes, and he will feel better. In that respect, the good friends are a good fence for health, and bad friends always bring diseases and sufferings.

When the will takes part, you can heal yourself alone. With the participation of will, you can stay for hours out, in the cold, in thin clothing, without catching a cold. Mentally, one can produce for himself a warm, magnetic garment, with which he will not tremble even in the sharpest cold. Without such a garment, without the participation of the will, no matter how well one is dressed, he may still be cold and take a chill.

If someone falls ill with rheumatism, he shall grasp it, shake it a little and start talking to it that it has mistaken its way and has to leave his body. If rheumatism is stuck somewhere in the shoulder, he shall direct it toward his elbow, then toward the fingers until he gets it out. Diseases are healed not only by medications, but also by thinking. The mind may expel any disease from the human organism. The mind is powerful.

If somebody suffers with fever, let him impose on himself the thought that he wants to get better, to devote his life to realizing a good, great work. Soon the idea begins to work in him and the fever will pass. If the idea gives a good result and he recovers, this shows that it has worked. Every idea, every virtue that can be realized, first improves the health.

Hindus have the following way of healing wounds: they gather prana from Nature and with the help of their minds they direct that prana to the ill place, which gets better within 20 minutes.

While living in the world of contradictions, you should know that you are under the law of suggestion. Neither mortals, nor immortals are free from that law. Having in mind this, you shall always keep in your mind positive thoughts and feelings if you want to get rid of many painful conditions, which are not yours. If you connect with someone, who suffers with pains in the leg, you will experience the same pain.

So, if you want to progress in life, apply the law of suggestion. When it comes to your family, you apply suggestion quite successfully. If it comes to you, you cannot profit from it. For example, if a friend of yours is discouraged and afraid that he will not pass the exam, encourage him, suggest to him that he will pass his exam and he will calm down. If you find yourself in the same situation, you cannot help yourself. So, the law of suggestion does not work for you. Apply this law to yourself, as well as to your friends, but always for the good, the positive in life. This law works everywhere. Consciously or unconsciously, animals and people use this law. As rational beings, you shall use suggestion in all cases in life: to heal, to strengthen your memory, to encourage, to withstand sorrows and sufferings, etc. The suggestion is a weapon, by which one can fight evil and the negative powers in the world. Contemporary people live in hell.

As disciples you must apply the laws of suggestion to influence yourselves in a positive way. If your memory is poor, work with suggestion to strengthen it. If someone likes to sleep a lot and cannot get up early, let him suggest every evening to get up in the morning, for example, exactly at 5 a.m. As a law, the suggestion makes sense when applied for acquiring something positive, for creating something good in human nature. Whether aware of it or not, all people and all animals use suggestion as a working method.

There are days and hours when suggestion affects humans harmfully. During that time people shall not suggest anything to each other. At such moments one should fence himself against suggestion in the same way, in which the military builds fortresses against enemies.

If a tumor appears in the abdomen or somewhere else, do not panic. This shows that excessive energy has accumulated at one place and it has to be chased out. You shall stimulate some of the surrounding healthy cells to expel that energy out. The mind shall be strong, focused and you will come to the natural state. If there is no other way, the disease may be eliminated by a surgery. However, with the help of a strong, concentrated mind, the tumor may disappear by itself. By suggestion, you may make even the strongest man fall ill. Through suggestion you can also take any tumor out of the body even for 24 hours. For three days you can take a tumor out by placing the patient in a magnetic sleep. Through suggestion any tumor can be removed. Everything depends on the mind.

While you are under treatment, you should use some magic formulas when the moon is emptying. For example, someone suffers with rheumatism. Let him does the following experiment: let him take half a kilogram of salt lumps (sea or rock) and put by one lump of salt in a vessel of clear spring water every day. He shall get up early, before sunrise, put a lump of salt in the water and say: "In the way salt melts in the water, in the same way my joints rheumatism will melt, i.e. will disappear." If it does not pass immediately, you shall do this experiment for two weeks while the moon is emptying. If rheumatism does not pass even after all this, let him do the same experiment at sunset and at Moon in the evening. While doing the experiment, he shall be careful that nobody watches him and never tell somebody until he gets a result. It is important for one to be persistent until he recovers.

If you are with a running nose, think about health. Repeat frequently the thought: "I am healthy" and soon you will get rid of the running nose. Healthy people often think of diseases and attract them. Do exactly the opposite - think about health, in order to attract and strengthen it and get rid of the disease. The rational, good, great in man is able to fight microbes that cause diseases. Apply the good and positive words and thoughts as formulas, with the help of which you may influence yourselves.

In order to understand if your faith has developed, i.e. whether you have enough will to apply an occult formula, the best experiment is the following: if sometimes you have a stomachache, test your will. Put your left hand behind on your back, and the right one – in front – on the abdomen, focus your mind and say the following formula: "Let the disease stop." If you do not remember that formula, say: "The disease has stopped."

How are TB cases treated today? They put them to bed without moving. They are under a special diet and nothing more. No. Let the patient be free to do whatever he wants. If he wants to rest, let him rest. If he wants to go for a walk, let him go for a walk. However, he shall start pronouncing every day the words: "I will recover". He shall gradually increase the number of repetitions of these words until he reaches 1000 - 2000 repetitions a day. Let him say these words 100 times during the first day, on the second day - 120 times, on the third day - 150 times and so on until he reaches 1000 - 2000 times. Every disease, every discouragement may be treated in this way. Thus, the heavy, dark atmosphere around the patient becomes cheerful, bright, and pleasant and he feels better and better. Then all healthy people will start to visit that man.

Let's say that you have a little difficulty. Your finger hurts and you cannot stand it. In order to heal yourself, or to be more precise, in order to be able to stand it, imagine that somebody has hammered a big nail in your hand. This bigger pain will replace the less one. If you can reproduce mentally that hammering of the nail into the hand, transformation of the pain will take place in your mind.

If you fall ill do not rush to call the doctor. Apply one, second, third method, concentrate your mind on the pain and say mentally several times the following: "I will recover." Sometimes you can say only ten times that you will recover and this will happen, but at other times, it will be necessary these words to be said thousands of times. No matter how many times you say these words, just do not discourage. Be persistent and you will get good results. In this way you can treat yourself and your friends.

A special atmosphere will be created around you if you know how to pronounce the words 'life', 'goodness', 'love', 'wisdom', 'spring', 'Christ', 'Spirit'.

If there is something wrong with your eyes, every night before falling asleep, you shall say: "When I open my eyes tomorrow, I will be better." One, who has faith, is capable of everything.

If there is a wart or lichen: a Bulgarian would go to a grocer, steal a lump of salt, because by stealing it, it will become positive, and he is also positive. And when the moon is emptying, he will surround the wart by the lump of salt and say: "Let the wart disappear in the same way, in which the moon is emptying and this lump of salt melts.", he throws the salt and the wart disappears. You explain that to yourself that the salt, as a channel, has attracted those flows in Nature, which support these warts.

You all want to be smart, healthy, good, clean - qualities that you can have if you know how to pronounce properly the word "Love". This word has a huge, powerful meaning, and it has also power in front of God and the angels and the people, only if you know how to pronounce it. It is a magic word that could revive even deceased. Everything submits to that word. It is a word that costs millions and billiards.

You shall make attempts. If ten people gather and focus their minds on an ill person, they can heal him by attracting positive and healing powers through their minds and prayers.

In order one to be able to cope with all energies in himself, he should study the law of concentration. By studying the law of concentration, one must attempt to focus his sight on an object without blinking. Do this experiment, starting from 1 minute and gradually increase the duration. It helps for strengthening of the eyes. Your mind should be focused during the experiment. During that time distraction of the mind is not allowed.

Attempt to heal yourself mentally with the participation of the will. If a furuncle appears somewhere on your body, apply mentally onion or another remedy on it and watch the result. If your mind is strong, the furuncle will disappear soon.

Somebody cannot sleep. If he is treated in a medical way, he will take a medicine and he will fall asleep, but he will not take a proper rest. If he wants to use the methods of occultism, he will say to himself: "I will go to bed now, I will fall asleep deeply and after 6 hours of healthy and nice sleep,

I will wake up." Modern medicine recommends quinine against fever, and occultism - to use your mind against the microbes of the fever: "I order you, microbes, to go out of my organism within 25 minutes, because I'm busy and I am off to work."

One may be a doctor to himself and heal without a knife. With the help of his mind, one may get rid of growths in the body. How? By moving them from one place to another. If the growth is internal, he can take it somewhere out. If it is external, it is easily treated.

By knowing the properties of warm and cold water, a person may also treat himself in a spiritual way. For example, instead of with the help of warm water, a person may treat himself through his mind, which causes the same expansion of the capillaries as the one, caused by warm water.

If you often direct your mind toward the roots of the hairs, for one year, you will achieve a lot: your hair will grow and strengthen. What causes thinning of the hair? It is a result of inner restlessness and lack of moisture in the organism.

If any of you falls ill, while he sleeps during the night, you may send good thoughts toward his subconsciousness that he will recover soon.

In order the hair to become black, you need to bring bright thoughts into your mind, beneficial feelings – into the heart, as well as to use nettles for half a year or for a year. All possibilities are hidden in the mind. It regulates the functions of the organs of the human organism. A negative thought may cause a number of painful states, and the harmonious one may eliminate these states.

If you are ill: imagine that the sun, the light fall on you like a shower and it seems you are in a sea of light, health, strength, power, goodness, as if you are immersed in God. If the disease is at a certain place, you shall say to the ill place: "Go out of here, I have work, I have to serve God, go away!" If the disease is all over the body, you shall say: "Go away from me." You shall make passes with your right hand from the top downwards, bringing your hand close to your mouth and shake it forward while blowing three times.

One, who understands the power of the circle, uses it for treatment. For example, he will draw that circle around the wart of his finger, he will take his hand away and after half an hour at most the wart will disappear. If you have a furuncle on your neck, draw a circle around it and concentrate your mind on it. The powers of the circle will begin to act on the furuncle and after a while the furuncle will disappear. In this way you will experience the power of your mind and the power of your faith. If you say you have faith, but you cannot treat even the smallest diseases, your faith is not strong. It is only in embryo.

I will give you a method by which to influence yourself if the liver is upset. Put your right hand in front of your abdomen with the palm facing the abdomen, and the left hand – on the wrist, again with the palm facing the body, and mentally pass the energies of the Sun toward the center of the Earth. After 10 - 15 minutes, your state will improve and you will become happy.

If the pulse is reduced to one beat, there is still a possibility of saving the patient. He may even spend three days with such a weak pulse. If the thoughts of his relatives are positive, the pulse will gradually accelerate. When the patient's relatives pray for him and have positive thoughts, they will save him.

Someone suffers with fever and in accordance with the advices of the doctors he has to use every day by 30 centigrams quinine. But this man is poor, he has in his pocket money only for bread. What should he do? Let him apply the law of autosuggestion and heal himself in this way. Let him go mentally to a pharmacy and buy 30 centigrams quinine. Then let him take, again mentally, that quinine and wait for a result. In this way he will recover twice more quickly than if he takes quinine for real. However, an intense thought is required for the experiment with suggestion. If the thought is not intense, one can go mentally ten times to the pharmacy without a result.

If I am a doctor, here is what I will do: I will prescribe a patient the various liquids and powders, which to be in a good interaction, and, as living elements, to enter his body. Their effect will start to show, but only on the condition that after each drug intake the patient says: "I will recover." In addition, I will engage a hundred poor people, I will pay them per five levs and I will tell them to go to that address, where there is an ill person, ask him how he is treated and tell him that he looks very well. After all of them have gone to see him, he will be healthy. However, the patient has given 100 levs for drugs, and I have given 500 levs to that one hundred people only to tell him by one good word for help.

Treatment Through Movement

Each our external action is an expression of an action that takes place in the spiritual world.

Any disharmonious movement in the physical world produces disharmony in the astral one. Any disharmony in the astral world also affects the mental one. Once the inner world balances, harmony in the movements of the external limbs will restore.

So, thoughts affect movements and movements affect the mind.

Every movement leaves cliches in the invisible world. And every cliche is an imprint that has its consequence. And that consequence, that result brings joy or sorrow.

By his movements, one regulates the energies of his organism. Movements jolt the air, whose vibrations are transmitted to the physical body through the doppelganger. The doppelganger of somebody is an antenna, through which he perceives impressions from the outside world. This is why the doppelganger wraps the human body and protects it from misfortunes. The better one regulates his doppelganger, the more correctly he perceives the impressions from the outside world. Knowing this, you have to adjust your antenna often.

When human movements are dictated by harmonious thoughts and feelings, they are always beautiful. The greater harmony exists in man, the more beautiful his movements are.

Arm movements affect the brain, the nervous system. If the movements during writing letters are correct, they affect favorably the memory, and hence, the development of the mind. They develop the mildness and stability of the human character. In general, all movements that you make determine your state and character.

Correct movements are those, during which the whole body takes part. The head shall be moved together with the legs, and the whole body shall move wave-like. If you walk in this way within mountainous areas, you will not feel any fatigue.

Rational movements help avoiding many painful conditions with humans. They regulate the nervous system, which bears the vital energies. The nervous system takes in the living powers of Nature. When the nervous system is in good condition, all body functions are carried out properly. When the nervous system of a person is not in good state, then no doctor is able to help him.

If you do not know how to step, how to walk, how to move, you will lose all conditions that you have gained from breathing, from the air and food. From the gait of a person you may see that he is a candidate for prison. See how animals and birds move. Your movements shall be beautiful, smooth, natural, and plastic. It is important with which leg you will get up in the morning. It is important with which leg you will start off to work, whether you move your arms slowly or fast, how you look. Lots of misfortunes befall you because they pay attention to these important matters. Through the movement of the arms, through touching, you may treat yourself, and you also may cripple yourself if you do not understand.

One must know how to stretch out his arm, how to stretch his legs. There are powers in the earth, which you will be able to take by stretching your legs and thus you will transform your state. If you are sad, desperate and if you know how to stretch the left arm and left leg, the earth will attract all the weight from your legs and you will feel a relief. Then you shall stretch your right arm and right leg.

All modern people, in general, step straight on the heel, then on the toes. That is why, while walking, there is thumping, resulting in spinal cord concussion and feeling of a back brain flow, because of which everyone is nervous. Therefore, you shall walk on your toes and you shall step lightly and smoothly. The light movement of the legs depends on the human mind. If your thought is materialistic, you will step in such a way on your feet that the earth will tremble when you walk. That shows that man is more connected to the center of the Earth than to the center of the Sun.

Toes are an angelic field of action, the bottom of the feet – a human field of action, and the heels - the animal field of action. One, who first steps on his heels, looks for the right of the strength. In the human world the right belongs to the one, who is rational and in the angelic world – to the one, who loves. The Divine world involves the right of all beings.

In the future, educated people shall adapt heels with springs so that when people step the movements will be facilitated by the contraction and expansion of the spring. Today's heels of shoes cause concussion in the spine at each step. As a result of that concussion, many people suffer with various disorders of the nervous system.

All movements are subject to certain rules and laws. For example, the human way of walking is also determined by certain laws. When a person starts off to somewhere, he first must put his right foot forward, and then the left one. Further, he must walk lightly on toes, and not first on the heel and then on the toes. It is a rule one to start off slowly, calmly and gradually to accelerate his gait. If he does so, finally he will walk easily, quickly, as if flying.

Aim at beautiful movements, at beautiful lines that affect you health well. By studying the beautiful lines and movements, you connect to the spiritual world, to the mind and feelings of spiritual beings.

Aim at pretty conscious plastic movements to rationally contact to the ebb and flow of the cosmic energy, i.e. to the flowing out and in cosmic energy. The exit and entry of the cosmic energy determine the health of people, as well as their thoughts and feelings.

If someone grips you by his left hand, he transfers feelings to you. If he grips you by his right hand, he transfers thoughts to you. However, if he grips you by his both hands, he transfers both feelings and thoughts to you. So, any movement, any change in Nature has its deep meaning.

If any of you falls ill, focus your mind on the disease and chase it out of yourself. If you cannot liberate in this way, you shall not lie down, succumbing to the disease, but go for a walk, move. Whatever the weather is - snow, rain - you should not be afraid. Diseases find a favorable soil with fearful people.

Paneurhythmy renovates and rejuvenates people. It treats not only diseases, but all mental and physical ailments. The entire human organism vibrates musically with it. And there are no diseases in the musical world, there are no interferences. Therefore, through these exercises, one goes out from the world of interference, disappointments, dissatisfaction, anxieties and troubles, and enters into a world of harmony. Those, who do these exercises consciously for one year, will be healthy, will get rid of many diseases or avoid them by raising the vital level of the organism.

Treatment Through Gymnastic Exercises

Exercises that you do are necessary, because more negative energy is gathered in half of your body and positive one - in the other half. During these exercises, the different energies in your body balance. When one is healthy, when one feels and thinks properly, the energies balance by themselves. But when a person is not healthy, Nature evokes the balancing of these energies by creating a certain disease and causing certain movements through this. When one is ill, he begins to writhe, to move, to get up and lie down, and energies balance in this way. If they are adjusted properly one recovers, if they are not adjusted properly, one leaves.

At gymnastic exercises, in order to contact the invisible worlds, you shall stretch your muscles. If your arms are loose, you will gain nothing. To perceive something, your arms are to be stretched.

You should know that with every move you connect to the flows of Nature. Once you stretch your arm and keep your mind focused, you are already in contact with these flows. And then, in each particular case, you may be connected both to the electricity of the Earth and to the electricity of the Sun. At each stretching of the arm, you may also have contact with the earth or solar magnetism. Magnetism, in general, is connected with prana, i.e. with the vital energy of Nature. Therefore, while stretching arms and legs and concentrating the mind, people use the vital energies of Nature and become healthy and strong. Natural powers cannot be used with loose arms.

During all exercises that you do, the mind shall present to attract natural powers that are necessary for you. If you move your arm mechanically, you use nothing. If you pass the mind through the forefinger, you will become more noble with dignity and merciful.

If you want to become fair, you should exercise the middle, Saturn finger.

For nobility and musicality, for sense of beauty, exercise the ring-finger, the fourth one. If you want to arrange your works well and have good relationships with the others, then exercise the little finger. If you want to gain something Divine, exercise the thumb.

The hand is a big wealth.

It is good, while making movements for regulating your organism, to accompany them by the vowels "a" and "o" - two powerful sounds. Rational movements regulate the nervous system, which bears the vital energies and takes in the living powers of Nature. When the nervous system is in good state, all body functions happen normally.

Taking your hands away from each other has a calming effect. When you move your hands against each other, the effect is the opposite of the above. So you will tell these opposing forces to move up.

I exercise. Raise both arms up and away from the sides of your body, palms down, at the height of the shoulders. Then the right arm is to be raised slowly up under an angle of 45° from the shoulder level, and the left arm is to be let down under an angel of 45° from the shoulder level and from this position, squat six times, and during that time, focus your mind on the front part of the brain.

The exercise is used for adjusting the front part of the brain.

II exercise. This exercise is like the first one, but the left arm is raised up under an angle of 45° from the shoulder level and the right one is to be let down under the same angle, at which you squat six times.

During that exercise, focus your mind on the heart. The exercise serves for regulation of the emotions.

III exercise. Bring both arms back, palms facing each other, and row forward, at which squat 6 times.

During that exercise, focus your mind on the spine. The exercise serves for regulation of the spine.

IV exercise. Raise the left arm up and forward to the east, and the right one downward, rotation of the body around the waist and swimming by arms. This exercise is also repeated 6 times.

While doing this exercise, focus your mind on the stomach. It regulates the stomach.

V exercise. Put your hands on your waist. Balance the body on the left leg, and the right leg is to be slightly raised to the right side, slowly forming a semicircle with it from left to right - 6 times. After that balance on the right leg and do the same with the left leg – again for six times.

During that exercise, focus your mind on the nervous system. It serves for regulation of the nervous system.

VI exercise. Raise both arms up and away from the sides of your body at the level of the shoulders and slowly raise up until fingers of both hands touch above your head. Lift the body on the toes and from this position slowly squat, at which arms are to be put back along your body. This exercise is to be done 6 times, too. It is a finish of the first five exercises. It is called a magnetic undressing and dressing: downwards - undressing, upwards - dressing.

Note: These exercises shall be done once a day. If they are done in the morning, it would be wonderful, at noon – nice, and in the evening - well. These exercises should be done very slowly and correctly, with well stretched arms and legs, if you want good results. Arm movement is for the development of the heart and chest. Concentration of the mind strengthens the mind. The execution of all exercises strengthens the will.

These exercises are one of the best occult exercises. However, take care they not to become like a loop for you, but benefit of them. Consider that you have known them once, and now you remember them.

I will give you now the following exercise with the pronunciation of the vowels "a" and "o". Put the palm of your left hand over the right one and bring it in this way to your shoulder. Then put your right hand over your left one and bring it again to the shoulder. Do this exercise for 10 days, every evening, before going to bed: 6 times with the left hand and 6 times with right one, by taking turns: left hand, right hand, etc. Start with the left hand.

Arm movements have a certain effect on all your organs and on your will. Let's say that sometimes you are excited. Do the following exercise with your hands: Put your hands in front of your chest, then up and away from the body on both sides, making slight wrist movements. Then put your hands in front of your mouth. By doing this exercise for 3-4 times and think on the three words, your discomfort will pass. This is a psychological treatment, psychological ventilation in man. You shall pronounce the words love, joy and gaiety. You shall have these words as keys.

The left hand is to be put freely on the knee. The right arm is to be raised up and away from the side of the body, horizontally, then forward, up, back in a circle, and down. That rotation of the arm is repeated several times. The same thing is to be done with the left arm and then with both arms together. Arms stop horizontally and go down.

This exercise is to be done during the week, in cases, when thoughts and feelings muddle up. When your thoughts muddle up, do the exercise only with your right hand, and when the feelings muddle up, do the exercise only with your left hand.

Arms up, well strained, end of fingers of both hands touched. Concentrate your mind and direct mentally the solar energy to pass through your hands, to flow throughout your body. At this position of the hands, say the formula: "I am in harmony with the animated Nature. Let God's goodwill flow through me!" Take hands down.

Left arm up, the right one - down. Try mentally to perceive the two flows. With your right arm you will perceive the flow from the Earth, and with the left one - the flow from the Sun. Remain in this position for 3 minutes. Try to feel the effect of flows along your arms.

Right arm up, left one – down, squatting, the fingers of the left hand touch the earth while you are saying the words: "I am connecting to the center of the Earth and evil, through my left arm, goes into that center." While getting up, your right arm remains up, and the left one – down, while you are saying the words: "I am connected to all intelligent powers, to all rational beings, Divine beings, as well as to God and let the Divine energy pass through my entire body." The squatting and the formula are to be repeated three times.

Formulas are to be pronounced mentally and with awe in the soul.

When a person gets into bad condition, during which his mind darkens and his feelings roughen, let him do the following exercise: let him put the palms of the hands against each other, ends of fingers touching. The left hand pulls along the palm of the right one to the end of the wrist, then straights in the position of a right angle with the right hand without interrupting the movement. The right hand is to be put on the left one (at that position both hands are horizontal). Now your right hand pulls, slides over the left one to the end of the middle finger. Finally, both hands are put with palms facing each other like at the beginning of the exercise. The same exercise is done with the right hand. If you do this exercise several times, all your bad conditions will disappear.

By giving this exercise, I want to draw attention to the following: slipping, hand raising and putting it over the other must be made without interruption. Nature does not like interruptions. By doing the exercise by changing hands, you polarize.

Left arm forward and slightly tilted, palm down. The right hand moves along the left arm. Start from the shoulder and go downward, while you are singing the exercise with the letter "Y" (the Bulgarian letter "Y" is pronounced [u] – transl. note). Then the hand goes down to the wrist, while you are singing the exercise with the letter "A" (the Bulgarian letter "A" is pronounced [a] – transl. note). Finally the hand goes up from the wrist to the elbow, while you are singing the letter "И" (the Bulgarian letter "И" is pronounced [i] – transl. note). The distance from the shoulder to the elbow is the material world, the physical world of the stomach. The zone from the elbow to the wrist is the spiritual world – the heart, and the wrist is the mental world – the mind. Then put your right arm forward, and the left hand is to be moved along it. Do this exercise for a week every morning and evening for ten times. This will improve the state of the stomach, the chest and the brain. You will treat yourself. One, who wants to be healthy, shall sing. If one is sad or does not feel well, he shall sing, too. Sing and praise God in your soul.

Right leg forward, easily bend the body to the earth, while imaging that you are lifting an enormous load. Do this exercise, gradually increasing the load until you reach 50 kg. By doing the exercise regularly, you will notice that your muscle strength has increased.

If you are able to lift 50 kg mentally and you will be also able to really lift it. Do this exercise when you do not feel well to see what powers you have.

In order your eyes not to weaken, you shall practice. There are exercises, which stir all eye muscles. If not exercised, eyes gradually weaken and lose their ability to see. When you go on an excursion, you want to reach the peak as soon as possible. This is not right. Go slowly and look up, left, right. Once the sun is up, stop for a while, to see how it rises and continue your way. If you are in a hurry, you will soon get old.

One of the reasons for weakening of the eyes is that they do not move. You move your neck when you want to see something and do not move your eyes. I would recommend an exercise that you can do in the morning and whenever you want during the day. Close your eyes and move them, look, as much as it is possible, up, then, as much as it is possible, down, as much as it is possible to the right, and as much as it is possible to the left. Repeat this several times very slowly. Then, during the day, when you want

173

to see something, do not twist your neck. The neck shall be still, and the eyes are to be moved –this will become the natural way of looking at things for you. This is the physical side. Inside is the following: if you make a mistake and do not fix it, then if you make a second mistake and do not fix it, third one, fourth one, you get used to that and your sight weakens. Another thing: You love someone and excuse his mistakes or you see them as too small ones. You do not love him, do not excuse his mistakes and you see them as too big. Third: eyes weaken as a result of worries, concerns, internal disharmonious states, or of dust.

Cold feet are the first condition of neurasthenia. It is good for neurotics and those, who often lose their temper, to remove their shoes from time to time and walk barefoot on sand or soft grass. In this way feet are in direct contact with the vital powers of the earth and tone. In the morning exercises, while lifting your arms up, you take in the solar energy and through legs – the earth energy. Hence, in the morning, you shall take in solar energies, and in the evening you shall do exercises to get rid of the energy, collected during the day. In the morning you will take in from the Sun, and in the evening you will give the excessive energy to the Earth.

Spiritual Healing

PRAYERS

When you pray, the image of God shall be in your mind.

A PRAYER FOR HEALING (of another person)

Omnipresent and almighty God, in the Name of the Lord, Who has spoken to Your servant, let Your cure come through us Your humble-servants, for the Glory of Your Name.

We thank you, that You have heard us. Only You are our Lord, besides You we have no other; You are the only One who can always heal. Your cure is health for the body and the soul.

Restore the mutual action between the mind and the soul, between the soul and the body. Turn the source of the heart for good and the powers of the body for useful work.

Let this our brother/sister by flesh, who suffers, accept Your mercy, so that we may always rejoice in the presence of Your Might.

Amen.

(The prayer is to be said each Wednesday, Saturday and Sunday at 7 and 9 a.m.)

A PRAYER FOR HEALING (of another person)

God almighty, You are our refuge. We glorify Your mercies forever. You have made covenant with Your chosen ones, because You have a sound and strong hand to give mercy to those, who know You in Your name.

Turn, God, Your eyes to the suffering brother / sister, give attention to his / her (-) sufferings and relieve them. We believe Your words, when you said: "Appeal to me and I will answer you, because I am your God, Who supports you and tells you: "Do not be afraid, I will help you! Do not be afraid, Because I chose you, I called you by name. You are not alone when you walk through the water, I will be with you when you walk through the fire, you will not be burned and the flame will not burn you. Do not be afraid in weakness, too, because I am with you!"

Now hear our prayer, God, pour over him / her (-) of Your abundant mercy!

Amen.

A PRAYER FOR HEALING (personal)

God, You are a source of life. Send in me Your life-giving power- the Spirit – to heal my mind, my heart, my soul, my will, and my body; to heal me from all psychic and physical diseases and sufferings, endow me with health, power and life, and develop in me gifts and abilities for being able to live, study and serve You.

Amen.

Healing Formulas

1. God, in You is all my trust. Help me, send me Your help. I promise to serve You, to dedicate my life to You.

2. God, from now on I will dedicate my whole life to You and I will work for You. Leave me on the Earth.

3. I, who serve God, want my body to be healthy, because it belongs to God. It is a cell from the Great Cosmos, so it must be healthy.

4. I believe in God out of me, I believe in God within me. My Father and I are one.

5. God is love, God is light, God is life, let His name be blessed now and ever.

6. God is Love, God is life, holy Love, most holy Love.

7. You put your left hand on the left side of the head and say willingly: "God, for Your glory, infuse and anoint health and life in my cells to serve You with joy and gaiety."

8. God, infuse purity in my body, in my Soul and in my Spirit.

There are two ways of treatment: old and new. Contemporary people usually take treatments in the old way by medicines, baths, etc. This way of treatment is slow and has a microscopic result. I also treat by this method. I do not treat people in the new way. Why? It is because they are not ready. The new way is a spiritual treatment. If I heal somebody in a spiritual way, when he is not ready to lead a clean life, he will make even more mistakes, and due to that he will cause to himself greater troubles in his life. For the one, who is ready, the spiritual treatment gives immediate results.

To treat somebody in a spiritual way, means the reasons for his disease to be found and he will never get ill again.

To take treatments in a Divine way means to change your life, to lead clean and sacred life.

When you get ill, first turn to God, then to your soul and finally to the doctor. You go in the opposite way and that is why you do not succeed.

The yeast and the milk compress are good healing methods, but temporary. If you want to be healthy, your heart and your mind shall direct to God, to the Sun, to all beings. The help for you will come from there.

Love is that cosmic power in the world, which may tone the human organism. Moreover, Love, in its low manifestation, is that power, which harmonizes all organs and gives an impulse to the human life. Love your body for not suffering. Pains show lovelessness.

When somebody gets ill, his first task is to turn to God with the request to give him a right way for treatment, to send him a person, determined for him.

If we work for God, for whatever we ask and even before asking for it, He will give it to us.

Each person, who takes treatments in the Divine way, cannot recover all at once, in a magical way, but gradually, with lots of crises.

When you come upon a suffering or an illness, do not be in hurry to call a doctor, do not philosophize, but turn your mind to God, to your intuition and you will get an advice from there what to do. Do not be afraid: diseases are a privilege to people; it is a privilege when you cannot eat and you have to go to bed hungry.

If somebody, who is ill, says to the doctor and his mother not to come to him, and he himself turns to God and promises that he will do God's will, that he is ready to sacrifice everything for God, and internal coup d'état will occur in him and his health will begin to restore. If he does God's will, he will recover; if he doubts and does not do it, he will go to the other world.

For each disease, pray sincerely for recovering.

A strong prayer is able to remove all human diseases.

Ordinary disciples may be treated in whatever way they wish, but occult disciples may be treated with the power of the prayer and of their minds.

It is enough to pray sincerely to God for the recovery of an ill person for Him to hear our prayer and answer it.

You will turn to God with a request once, twice, three, four times to give you whatever you need. Then God will say to the Sun to satisfy your needs. If you are ill, you will recover.

If you get seriously ill, turn to God in an earnest honest prayer. Say: God, help me in this difficult hour to get rid of the disease to serve You with joy. I want to dedicate my life to Love, to do Your will." Any answer to your prayer shows that you are connected to God.

The prayer helps only when you work for God. Then God will also work for you.

If your prayer is sincere and the vibrations are strong, it will come out of the atmosphere of the Earth and go to its place. It means "close to God".

If your prayer is not sincere, it will be far from God.

One may also pray with his own words, besides the given prayers.

The greatest doctor is inside you. When you get ill, you shall say: "I will live. I have a lot of work to do. I have done nothing so far, I have to live and when I finish my job, I will depart then." You will say so to the higher beings and they will help you, they will not fire you. And the psalmist says: "Do not take me, God, at the half of my days, to gain what I want, to understand Your law. To correct my life and live as long as I should."

If you are sad, ill, depressed, say the word "aum" often, even if you do not understand the meaning, "aum" is a word of the Spirit, your spirit understands it, and that is enough.

At a period of examinations, of difficulties and sufferings say: "Fir-fur-fen, Tao bi aumen" – "Without fear and darkness, with life and light. On to infinite love."

Love heals even the incurable diseases. If you suffer with rheumatism, warm water, wash your feet and groins, and say: "In the name of God's Love, rheumatism will leave me." By calling Love, every disease, every difficulty disappears. They are provided as a condition for focusing, for a link between the human soul and God.

If you get ill, do not be afraid, but put your hands on the ill place and say: "This is an eternal life to know You, the only true God and Christ, whom You have sent."

Love is a powerful force that cures all diseases. If you pronounce the word "Love" correctly, you can be treated. For example, if you suffer with rheumatism in your legs, say deep inside yourself with faith and trust in the Great: "God is Love and in Love diseases do not exist." If you say these words 2-3 times, the pain will disappear and you will stand on your feet as healthy as you were once. Do not wait for someone to help you from outside. If you expect an external help, you solve problems mechanically.

If you are irritated by a great contradiction, do the following exercise: with the first three fingers of the right hand grip the left forefinger. The middle finger of the left hand touches the left thumb and you say: "Through God's Love everything is achieved (three times). Through God's Love, which is manifested in the human heart, everything is achieved." (Three times).

Mystical healing:

You shall forgive everyone, see the good in everyone, love everyone, send them all your love, ask God to send his blessing upon them. In this way you will know God's Love to you and feel peace and joy.

Sacred healing, mental healing:

1. First I will imagine the Sun, the light. I will think on them. I will imagine that the sunrays fall like a shower upon me and it seems that I am in a sea of light, health, strength, power, all good in God, etc.

2. I will think on why the disease came. I will raise my thought, pray to God to show me what my diversion from God's law is.

3. The Good Prayer.

4. The Sacred Formula of the disciple: "Gracious and Holy and Gentle God, manifest the light of Your face to do Your will." Formulas are spoken in your mind with awe in the soul. (This treatment is successful only at sacred disposition of the spirit.)

"In the name of my Master, who shows me the way to God, in the name of his holy name, you shall go out of the ill place, I have to serve God, go away!" (If the pain is at a certain place, I will say: "From the ill place." If it is all over the body, I will say: "Go away from me!"). At the last words (go away), passes are to be made with the right hand on the ill place from top to bottom and then approach the hand to the mouth and then shake it off forward while blowing. This is done three times.

One, who believes, will be healthy. Faith is the link between God and the human soul.

Faith is a power that constantly grows – turns into knowledge. By faith one may recover from any disease.

To clean from all sediments that are in the organism and get rid of these acids that corrode you, focus your mind on God.

If you want God to heal you, you shall completely trust Him. If you turn to God, no doubt shall exist in you. Put your love, your faith in the First Cause of things and think of nothing else. When you pray to God, get up and walk. If you believe, you will get well. The least hesitation is able to impede your recovery.

If your leg hurts, you shall tell the rheumatism: "I give you seven days for you to leave my leg", nothing more. Say this and forget it. If the rheumatism disappears, your faith is strong, if it does not disappear, the faith is weak. Christ said: "You all, if you ask, in my name, you will be." I believe in the power of faith, which may heal all diseases. While attempting to heal by the power of faith, you will not take any drugs and external means. You will rely on the power of faith. It will be your point of support. Our health depends on faith. The development of our minds depends on faith. The condition of our hearts depends on faith. Our public position depends on faith. Even future depends on faith.

The thing that heals is Nature, and not humans. The fact that someone prayed and recovered through a prayer is not quite right. When he prayed, he was an assistant. Christ, who knew the law, said: "Let it be according to your faith." Let it be the way you believe. Faith is a factor.

There is no disease that does not submits to faith. When you recover, do not rush to tell people how you have recovered. When some time passes, you may apply the same method to the others, too. If you tell people how to heal before seeing results, the disease will come back again.

Not all blind people may be able to look again and not all lames may be able to walk again. Only those, who are clean in their thoughts and desires and only the one, who is free from the bonds of his past, may see and walk again.

If the person you want to treat in spiritual way, is not related to causal world, you will not cure him. Faith is necessary for a result. Children, who have no faith, are treated by their parents with their magnetism – a mother will treat her daughter, and the father - his son.

While the patient has doubt, he just puts obstacles in the way of his treatment. Once he stops doubting, the disease goes away. It is a law: what one thinks, he holds that. If he stops thinking about that, it loses its power. A thing is powerful for somebody if he believes in it.

Imagine that in your shoulder or in your arm rheumatism occurs. What would you do? If you have understood the new methods, you must turn to God with gratitude that He has sent that rheumatism to teach you something. Praise God, the saints, the angels, the good people all over the world and when you connect to them, you will not notice the disappearance of rheumatism.

Everyone should strive for unity of consciousness as a method of treatment, as a method of work on himself. No matter from what disease you get ill, it is enough you to restore the unity of your consciousness to get up from your bed healthy and cheerful. The higher powers of the consciousness direct towards your organism and begin to influence it until a twist occurs in your body as a result of which all energies begin to flow up, begin to move to the opposite direction. In this situation, foreign substances in the organism that cause diseases disappear right way.

If somebody in whom the divine consciousness works goes to an ill person, it is enough to put his hand on the head of the patient for him to recover

The Holy Scripture is not alive word, but its content introduces vitality in humans. Turn that energy into life and the patient will recover. Put your hand on the head of a patient with good thoughts and love and see how this will affect his health.

If someone falls ill, but does the will of God, there is no need for him to look for doctors. As long as he is harmony with the Divine laws, he will send his thoughts to all good people on the Earth and up in heaven and he will recover – they will perceive his thought and come to the aid.

There are two methods for purification of the human blood - through thoughts and through feelings. Feelings are cleaned by giving. By giving love, the human heart expands. The wider one's heart is, the more easily it is cleaned. If someone is poor and cannot give, he shall do mental exercises, imagine that he has a great wealth and give everything to the poor and suffering people. Life always brings conditions to people for cleaning of the heart. You may give material things, as well as cordial and mental ones. The cleaner human thoughts and feelings are, the more his blood is clean. Pure blood brings health and joy.

When the human body becomes ill, he may be treated through the truth. While he does not like the truth, you can never be physically healthy. If you begin to love truth, you will restore your health and your body adopts the relevant fragrance. If deep down in his soul a person decides to love the truth and if he absolutely excludes the lie from himself, no matter what disease has reached him, he may be healed.

If you have an ache somewhere, e.g. stomachaches, if I were you, I would do the following: The day when your stomach begins to hurt, cook a nice meal and call a poor man to treat him well. You shall not eat, but watch and pray silently during that time. You may call a child or several strong people. It is all the same. The only important thing is to feed someone. I do not know anybody, who had a stomachache and invited somebody for that reason.

The day when you catch a cold in the head, do one microscopic good to the most miserable person, whom you find, and you will see what will happen to the cold. If you have a headache or a stomach ache, do the same.

Bright thoughts and lofty feelings regulate the nervous system, blood circulation, breathing, and from there - digestion.

Treatment by Plants

There are plants that treat the most dangerous and hardly treated diseases. One, who does not know them, suffers. Therefore, we say that people suffer because of their ignorance. Study plants and their healing properties.

There are herbs that replace even the most prominent surgeons – only if you know which they are and how to apply them, you will be able to help yourself.

Explore the magical power of plants. They have huge hidden powers.

You may treat yourself through their leaves, roots, flowers, but if you do not understand them, they cause misfortunes against their will. It is enough you to begin to sweat and to lie down close to the roots of a plant or a tree, e.g. a nut tree, to see what there is in plants. They love water and by pulling out water they also pull out juices of life. Never fall asleep in the shade of a tree. It is not a problem if the shadow is dapple.

In May and June, on beautiful sunny days, early in the morning gather herbs, dry them, and then put them in glass jars, covered, to stay a little more under the sun. A little tiny leaf of grass or a flower, if needed, is the best doctors.

Take a little yarrow, drink a little and your cough will go away. Summer time you all shall gather yarrow. There shall be yarrow at each home - white and yellow yarrow, and one that cannot be treated by his will to drink these herbs. You shall also have blue gentian. Gather from it. They are magnetic plants that help. Gather some thyme, green leaves of strawberries. They are also healing. Gather small camomile. You will have a whole pharmacy of glass vessels. And these leaves and flowers, when you put them in vessels with covers, put them in the sun to bake, to take some more energy from the Sun. Do not put them in humid places.

It is enough to take colt's foot and you will rejuvenate. But you shall know on what day of the year to take it, whether when it blooms and, in general, during which month of the year. In my opinion, it is best to take it when positive powers in it balance. One must come upon that moment when the colt's foot is in the state of self-satisfaction and ready to give, to help. This also concerns all other plants. Then one should go out early in the morning or at sunrise, when the sky without a single cloud. If there is even a small cloud, the medicine spoils. If you obey all these conditions, these moments, then you will pick one flower and put it in a glass vessel. If you know this art, when to pick that flower, you will experience a big thrill when you get close to the colt's foot, because it will rejuvenate you and happiness will come to you. In the morning, at sunrise, you will pick the flower and put it in a glass vessel. I agree with you that it is hard for people to come upon exactly such a combination, such a day. The day must not be hazy. There will come a day when this knowledge will be reached, but this can only be achieved through Love. Love is to be penetrated in man and rule him. I mean the sublime Love. The aim of the Sublime Divine Love is to restore the juvenile state of the entire mankind.

If your stomach aches, boil a little yarrow. To get rid of the cough, boil a little blue gentian.

If my friend has troubles, suffers, I will tell him to take by three fingers a little flowers of wormwood, put it in a pot for five minutes to popple and every day for 10 days to drink a cup of wormwood and he will improve his state at 75% for sure. He shall drink it without sugar.

If you have a toothache, boil walnut leaves and rinse your gums with this water.

Note all plants, of which the corollas of the flower are five. Their effect is laxative. So, the number 5 is a label, showing some properties.

If an entire year you eat nettles, your hair will become black.

When you do not feel well, take on the tip of a knife ash of burnt maple, put it into a cup of hot water and when it settles down, drink the water.

Through flowers, plants, fruits, trees, people heal themselves, connect with their magical powers. In every garden there shall be a bed of garlic, onion, and parsley. Their healing properties are enormous.

Flowers are remedies for many diseases. For example, the clove treats certain nerve diseases. The rose cures other diseases. The crocus, snowdrop, dahlia and all flowers cure known diseases and at the same time maintain and educate respectively each flower and virtue.

Flowers have a healing power. It is well one, who is anemic, to grow red flowers. The red contains a magnetic power that energizes the nervous system. If someone has no faith, he has to grow blue flowers.

To be healthy, plant flowers in pots or in your garden, and grow them. Also plant fruit trees and vegetables, study them in order to benefit from the powers that they have. Walk barefoot during the summer for 1-2 hours along the grass and stones.

You may recover from your indisposition if you have a flower garden with various flowers, if you have an orchard and a vegetable garden and take care of them. If you are anemic, you shall grow cherries. If your faith is weak, you shall take care of cabbage. These are external formulas for strengthening, for energy, for peace.

Fragrant substances, which the flowers of the carnation have, may be used as a remedy, but till a certain dose. The rose and carnations shall be smelled from afar.

If your eyes are weak from anxieties and troubles, look at yellow flowers.

MAGNETIC TREATMENT

There is a magnetic school, in which patients are treated through passes. During that magnetic treatment, when the patient begins to take treatments, his state first worsens, he passes through a terrible crisis, and then an improvement comes; then another crisis - again improvement, again crisis, again improvement. The crises decrease and when the last crisis comes, the disease will go back.

When a doctor treats a patient in a magnetic way, above all, he must be strong and in good moods, not to succumb to the ill states of the patient that is so close to him. The patient will also take some of the energies of the doctor, who is healthy, after which a struggle occurs in his organism, at the end of which conscious life awakens in the cells of the body. Then, after receiving the necessary building material, the cells begin to weld the ill places in the body.

Some doctors make of passes as a method for regulating the energies of the organism, but one, who undertakes to this method, should be a clean man. Clean thoughts and desires are good conductors of living powers of Nature.

Usually the black lodge hypnotists make passes from top to bottom. The disciple must make movements, i.e. passes to the sides, conversely to those of the black lodge. Every move you make has its deep meaning and affects you.

There are people, who may treat in a magnetic way, but there is a risk of introducing a disease of the one, who treats, together with the positive things introduced. For example, a person has a physical illness, but during his magnetic healing he loses this disease and gains a negative quality. He becomes doubtful, loses his faith in God, which have had before.

When you put your hand on the head of somebody, you should know if you take or give something. If you take something, you shall know if it will be of benefit to you. If you give, you again shall know if the one, who receives something, will benefit of it. In order to understand and use well both giving and taking, one shall thank. The energy that flows through the one, who gives and through the one, who takes is Divine and it is taken into account. It cannot and should not be spent in vain. Nature is a great system of energy and keeps an accurate account of everything that is spent. It also controls the results, obtained during the spending of that energy.

The interruption of the consciousness happens always when the doppelganger leaves the body. In order the doppelganger to return to the body, several passes along the spine of the person shall be made.

While treating someone, during all the time you need to be in a prayer, be connected to God. Only in this way treatment will be successful.

In five minutes one may modify his state from bad to good. It is enough a magnetizator to pass his hand along the left side of your body to change your state into good one. If he passes his hand along the right side – the good state will be changed to bad. In order you to persuade a person something, the words that you use shall contain power. Only one, who is enlightened, may use suggestion and hypnotism, because he knows the power of words and when to use them.

When the right side of a man is positively electrified, he must find a friend, whose left side has the opposite electricity, in order both types of electricity to neutralize each other. One of them has to put his left hand on the right side of the other, and he - his right hand on the left side of the head of his friend, and they will not notice how they will gain good states. This can be also achieved only by holding hands.

When someone is very excited and feels that his solar plexus is not in good state, the most natural movement for him will be he to put his right hand on the solar plexus, under the pit of the stomach, palm downwards, and his left hand on his waist, palm outward . In this position of the hands one feels calming of the nervous system. When one puts his hand on the solar plexus in this way, he passes the excess brain energy through his hands and calms down. The palm of the right hand is a conductor of negative, pacificatory energy, and the upper part of left arm is a conductor of positive, stimulating energy. These energies, gathered at one place, calm you.

Put your hand on the patient's head with all your love and see how it will affect his health. Your love and good will toward the patient will become a powerful living force.

I would like you to have such a will, to put your hand on the wound and after 20 minutes it to disappear. A person with a strong will may do that. Why? Because he may concentrate prana from the air and direct it to his wound.

If a stout person suffers with a stomachache, let him call a close friend – a thin, but healthy person - and ask him to put his right hand on his solar plexus and hold it there for 5-10 minutes and the stomachache will disappear. And if a dry person suffers with a headache, let him find a stout, healthy man and ask him to hold his forehead at temples with one or both hands and the headache will disappear. In this way people may help each other.

The remedy against anger is to find a friend, who is negative and passive. Ask him to put his left hand on the right side of your head and you will see that after a short time all the excess energy from you will go into his hand and you will be relieved.

If someone falls on the ground and breaks his leg or bumps somewhere hard, in order the pain to pass, he shall slowly begin to massage the spine or elsewhere. If every day someone massages your spine, each pain that you have will pass. This shows that some areas of the organism contain within itself hidden vital energy that heals ill places. When the activity of that energy is evoked, it and its effect immediately show up.

If you have a stomachache, put both hands on the stomach and after 45 minutes you will not have pains. This happens in accordance with one law: the cosmic flow of love passes through the left hand, and through the right one – the cosmic flow of wisdom, of knowledge.

Let us assume that you are excited, that someone has made you angry, that you have lost balance. Lift your hands up and do the following: slowly raise both hands above your head and gently touch with them in front of the whole body down past your head and then shaking off (magnetic pouring). This exercise can be done up to 3 times a day.

If you do not feel well put your left hand on the eyes, touching the nose. Then slowly, gently pass round the mouth and put it down. You shall do this three times. Then pass the second finger of the right hand above his nose, again three times. That exercise shall be done consciously.

I will give a method, by which to influence yourself if the liver is upset. Put your right hand in front of your belly, palm facing the belly, and the left hand on the waist, again palm facing the body, and mind and pass the energies of the Sun to the center of the Earth. If this method does not help, please, turn in your mind to the One, Who has harmony in himself. To understand what the state of your liver is, look what color your face is, the light of the eyes and their vitality. If the eyes are lively, the face is also lively.

187

The eyes of people shall be focused; they shall not to wander in different directions.

When you do not feel well and do not know what to do, grip one by one, with your right hand, first the thumb, then the forefinger, the middle finger, the ring finger and the little finger. Then watch what changes occur in you.

Thumb is the Divinity in man. It must constantly move. If you fall ill, move your thumb! Fingers are antennas, through which man communicates with the spiritual world.

When you do not feel well, do an experiment with your thumb to see what powers it has. Stroke the top part of your thumb, starting from the third flank and go toward the nail. Then stroke the base of the thumb, the mount of Venus and watch if the discomfort will disappear. If during the first stroke the discomfort does not disappear, stroke it some more times.

It is enough to put several times your middle finger, well washed in clean water in order the water to take the energies that flow out from it. If you drink that water, your state will improve. These are a special kind of drugs that are hidden in the man himself.

To restore your health, you have to pull your fingers several times a day. First you will grip the thumb. If you do not recover, grip the second finger. If the disease is serious, you shall grip one by one all fingers and toes. By pulling your fingers several times a day, for ten days, you will completely recover or at least your state will improve.

Those people, in whom the respiratory system is not well developed, for its strengthening, they may use the following method: a short massage of the bone behind the ears for increasing of the life.

When a person has been ill for some time and has lost some of his vital energy, let him grip, from time to time, by two fingers, the lobe of the ear and stretched it slightly down. Do this when you feel depressed, too.

If somebody suffers with neurasthenia or is depressed, let him go for a little walk to the nearby garden or forest, turn to the east and lean his back on a thick tree (elm, oak or pine), put his right hand on the chest, and the left on – on his back. In a little contemplation, let him start thinking about the impact of the tree and after 5, 10, 15 minutes or an hour at most his mood will change. He will draw some power, an exchange between his magnetism and the magnetism of the tree will take place and he will feel some improvement. He shall go to that tree once, twice, or three times and it will cure him. This is a natural way of healing. In old days people treated themselves in this way.

When you lean on trees in order to heal yourself, it is better to remain in that position from 5 to 30 minutes, you back touching the tree, and the head a little tilted.

At noon, when the sun is strong, you may sit down on stones. They have adopted solar energy and they heal.

If you sit down on a stone, you shall remain in such a position for about 1-2 hours. Good places for healing are the stony ones, because while you are sitting on stones, you are getting magnetized. They should not have edges, because the magnetic powers flow out through them. The stones are especially healing in September.

Treatment Through Precious Metals and Precious Stones

Precious stones and metals have a positive effect on human health. Gold has the strongest influence, because it has a magnetic power.

Gold is a symbol of the spirit - crystallized sunlight.

There is consciousness in the gold, not in the gold itself, but in those, who are masters of gold. If you love these masters, their hearts open and they will give you what they have, but first you need to meet them.

Gold is a stored solar energy that Hindus call prana, and human health depends on it. Prana is contained in the Sun. Therefore, it is recommendable for people to go out early in the morning to take a large amount of prana.

Gold is the best conductor of life, prana, and vital energy. One, who has more gold in his blood, enjoys a longer life. If gold in somebody is little, he is ailing. Spiritual science has formulas, through which gold is attracted.

As good conductors of warmth and electricity, gold and silver may be used as remedies. Give one gram of pure gold to somebody, who does not feel well, and see how his unwellness will disappear. The same concerns silver. Pure silver cleans like the Moon, and gold is considered a symbol of life. Silver takes out impurities, and gold brings life to one, who is depressed.

Take one gram of pure native gold, put it in ten grams of water and let it for a few days in the sun. If you are not well, take ten drops of that water and the discomfort will pass. If you are ill, take ten drops of that water. In general, no matter what you have experienced, treat yourself by that water.

When treated, put a gold coin in the water to stay awhile and then drink from it by one teaspoon a day.

Everyone has a certain amount of gold in him. And he externally may be so rich as much organic gold there is in his blood.

Gold may heal neurasthenia - a gold coin is to be put in clean water to stay for several hours. Microscopic particles of gold will dissolve in the water and it becomes healing. It will soothe a nervous person. Wearing gold jewelry is not senseless. I advise you to always have a gold coin with you.

Silver heals. If you have any pain, take pure silver, put it in water for 24 hours, and after that drink from that water from time to time.

By speaking about the properties of gold, I mean the primary gold that has come out with the first ray of light and passed through the true sun, then through the dark, then through our one and come, together with it, to Earth. That gold contains four valuable qualities that bring the suns through which it has passed. It may be said for that gold that it is a bearer of life. If someone reaches the gold, while he is passing through the dark sun, he is capable of killing somebody. When someone wants to live good, holy life, it shows that he has reached the gold, which has gone through four transformations. That man understands the properties of gold and uses them for his great works and achievements. When gaining such gold, one must understand the good that is in it, perceive it and introduce it in his organism.

Precious stones are bearers of life. If someone, who is ill, has a diamond, he will recover. Not only precious stones, but precious metals also bring life, so I would recommend that you bring at least one golden ring or another golden object, which a conductor of life. Rich people love gold, but do not know how to use it. They keep it closed in safes and become its slaves. In the future, those, who will marry, take gold from their blood. To make a golden ring from your blood for your beloved is a real and conceptual marriage.

The precious stone decomposes light in a special way. Everyone may be healed in that light. So, it is better one to wear golden rings with precious stones. Not all stones have a beneficial effect on the human organism and not each precious stone is healing for all people. There are some stones, whose vibrations are not in harmony with the vibrations of the organism of a certain person, thus producing disharmony.

The precious stone refracts light correctly, completely different from the ordinary stone or glass. If you direct a precious stone to a wound, the light that it refracts will heal the wound. A scientist refracts in a special way the sunlight in his mind and may heal with this light. An ordinary person refracts the light not very well and therefore cannot help neither himself, nor his neighbors.

The precious stone has a special life and a special healing effect, if you know how to connect to its energies.

Precious stones also may fall ill. They lose their luster then. They recover if they are worn by a healthy person in good state. Ordinary stones also may get ill.

Precious stones, amulets, talismans help against the bad influence of the stars.

It is good for one to have at least one golden ring with a precious stone and put it, every morning, consecutively on all fingers and say: "I want to unlock the Divine in me, to be noble, to be fair, to be musical, aiming at the beautiful, and treat people well." There is great power in precious stones.

Rings may be worn on the first finger, on the second and third finger of one of the hands, then you will put them on the other hand.

Other Methods

If you have cold in the head or cough, breathing is difficult, because the capillaries have contracted. To restore circulation, the patient should be massaged with olive oil or camphor spirit.

If you have caught a cold, have you back massaged to improve blood

MASTER BEINSA DOUNO

circulation, capillaries to expand, and normal state of the organism to be restored.

If you are depressed, draw 100 vertical parallel lines and the discomfort will disappear. You will also strengthen the will in this way. Parallel lines are a sign of rationality. If you keep one and the same distance between them, you adjust to a rational life.

A violin, which has been played by prominent masters and virtuosos orchestras, is healing. It is enough for someone ill to touch it to heal instantly. It has higher vibrations, so it sounds nice and harmoniously.

Nervous people shall go on excursions. The mountains have a healing effect on the nervous system. Nervous people shall do physical exercises and treated through music. They shall not drink cold water and they shall eat less.

If two bees sting a person, they will help him against rheumatism, but if one hundred bees sting him, they will kill him.

For strengthening of the eyes, it is well to go out in the evening in stormy dark nights and spend out in the open for about an hour. In this way eyes strain and more blood comes to them.

To enhance your sight, go out after midnight, from midnight to 1 a.m., when the sky is starry to watch the stars. It is also good to go out in a dark, stormy night. This experiment is also for strengthening of the nervous system. The experiment will have a result, if you are not afraid.

If you get angry, take a deep breath, exhale and count from 1 to 100, if the anger is still there, take a deep breath again, exhale and count from 1 to 200 and to 300 - this is one method for regulation of the energies. If you do not apply that method, then drink (again for the anger) one cup of hot water in swallows. Anger develops warmth in people, and similar is treated with similar.

If you your spirit is tired, put your hand on your forehead. Your status will change in ten minutes. You may write numbers, draw straight lines, draw pictures. Draw a triangle, paint it red, blue and green, and after 3-4 minutes your mood will improve. If you are crabbed, unsatisfied, angry, go out in the forest and cry, scream against trees, stones. You will get ozone and it will pass. You can then laugh at what you did in the forest. You shall draw powers from Nature.

When you want to bring into your character more softness, for a year, three times a day (in the morning, at noon, and in the evening) caress your palms. If you want to bring more firmness, courage, bravery, caress the upper part of your hands.

For Children

On pure or impure matter, whichever mother has, depends what a child will be born – a saint or a villain. In the process of conception and creation of the child, the Divine is not present yet - it is a lower process. The Divine comes afterwards, after the birth of the child, when it is differentiated as matter and spirit. While it is only matter, there is nothing sublime.

When does someone die, when is a house demolished? It happens when it is not done according to the rules of Nature, as well as to the engineering requirements. If a child is conceived in unfavorable conditions, he may not live long.

The first impact comes from the mother and father. Mother affects child while it is still in the womb through her thoughts, feelings and actions. The food of the pregnant woman has not less influence on the development of the child, as well as the food given to the child after its birth. The spiritual life of the mother depends on what the child will be.

A mother, who wants to give birth to a good, rational, and healthy child should constantly keep that idea in her mind. A mother will give birth to such a child what she wants. It depends on the mother what her children will be.

Any woman, who wants to become a mother, to have a child that to serve God, shall not allow even one bad feeling in her heart, even one evil thought in her mind, even one bad deed. She shall never be tempted in her soul.

During pregnancy, women are extremely responsive, so it affects the child. Knowing this, she shall avoid meeting people, who have physical or mental disabilities.

Vices of parents are transferred to the child through blood. While living in this world, there are a number of conditions for transferring weakness of this world and for accepting them.

A man and a woman, who have lived in love and purity, give birth to healthy children, viable, full of love.

While a woman is pregnant, she should keep in her mind clean desires and clean thoughts in her heart in order not to taint the blood of her child. If she transfers her impure blood to her child, the child will bear the consequences of that blood during its whole life. You will then wonder why your child is ailing with a yellow face.

During her pregnancy, a woman must eat properly, with good, harmonious state of the mind. She shall never eat if she is not in the most favorable conditions. She shall breathe deeply, think and feel right. In such a state women are highly sensitive and perceptive, with great imagination. Her relatives and she herself should create views, occupations and most sublime pleasures. She shall go for a walk at sunrise, look at the beautiful pictures of the rising sun, then she shall go for a walk in gardens while beautiful fragrant flowers are blooming and fine fruit trees grow. Wherever life grows and develops, its sense is there. Purity, both physical and spiritual, is a needed condition for a pregnant woman. You cannot find a greater purity than the one in Nature. For this purpose, she must visit clean springs and rivers, whose waters serve as a mirror of her life. Quiet, pleasant nights with a sky dotted by countless fluttering stars are also irreplaceable pictures for a woman, who is a future mother.

In the future, while still pregnant, woman will have to teach the child how to eat. Food accepted by a pregnant woman and the way it is accepted greatly influences the child that would be born. Food creates people. It raises or lowers them.

The greatest evil for modern women is miscarriage. Statistics show that in New York, in 1905, one hundred thousand miscarriages took place. It is not allowed for someone to miscarry a child neither from the mind, nor from the womb, nor from the heart if one wants to be a Christian. If a good thought comes to you, you say: "I will throw it away." You will throw, but then you fall ill. It is not a sin that you have had a bad thought, but the sin is to miscarriage. There are already idiots in the world. Bad thoughts that torture you are those children, those thoughts, those desires that you have miscarried once and now they impede you in any endeavor of yours. So, from now on, do not miscarry and pray God to forgive you for the bad use of all good thoughts and wishes, of all your children you have killed.

Women, who want to get rid of pregnancy, do not know that any violence on themselves bear not only physically, but also spiritual consequences.

Miscarriage is ten times more dangerous than childbirth, because Nature is rational and every woman is compensated. She renovates with every birth. She becomes wiser, and the one that miscarries, loses heart and organic powers.

After a birth, the internal connection between a child and a mother continues, although in another way. A child that was carried by its mother, but not breastfed, loses something very precious. There is a connection between the ether doppelgangers of the mother and of the child. That is why the child should not live away from the mother till its 14th year. The milk of the mother is very important for the child. When the child touches the breast of the mother, it is influenced not only by the milk, but also by the magnetic power that flows alternately from the left and right breasts of the mother. The effect will not b e the same if the child is breastfed by another woman. A power comes out of the mother, which nobles the child. When a mother breastfeeds her child, she should be in good moods and not angry.

A child that was not breastfed by the mother cannot become a person, nor a genius, nor a saint. When a mother breastfeeds her child three years on the run, she should live a pure life, without any negative thoughts. She shall be quiet and calm. Nothing would disturb her peace. There are rational powers in the mother's milk that could not be found in any other food.

A mother must not only give birth to a child, but she shall also breastfeed it. That milk shall be incorrupt. So many mothers have poisoned their children with their bad milk. If she is angry several times a day, a few hours after that she will poison her child.

If the mother is healthy, the more your child sucks, the better. Children, who have sucked for two or three years, are healthier. A healthy person is also good.

Every mother should know how to treat her children. Mother must give first aid. The first task of a mother is to give castor oil to an ill child. Then it shall drink several cups of warm water, and then the mother shall cook a vegetarian potato soup for the child. This is the first aid for every patient. You ask why you should drink hot water. It is very simple. While eating, fat deposits remain along the walls of the stomach and intestines that impede proper digestion. Hot water dissolves them and regulates the processes in the stomach and intestines.

195

If the child is anemic, give it more pears and cucumbers. If its character is a bit rough, feed it with apples. If he lacks noble qualities, feed it with cherries. Give children only fresh food, mainly fruits.

The first task of the future education of children will be the condition of the digestive system to be controlled. A healthy digestive system provides a normal brain system. If those two systems are in good working order, the function of the respiratory system is also good. These are the three main systems that regulate human thoughts and feelings. If they work well, thoughts and feelings of people will be expressed properly.

The child that eats bread, baked in the embers, has a hundred times bigger opportunity to become a distinguished professor than the child that eats cakes, chocolate and sweets.

When your children are ill, it is good the bone behind their ears to be massages - there is a living center. These massages make the organism elastic and durable.

If a child has been ill for a few months, the first thing that shall be done after its recover is to be bathed and dressed in new clothes. The old clothes, in which it has spent the illness, shall be burned. Old clothes are penetrated with negative states and therefore they shall be burned, and you shall not give them to poor. New clothes shall be given to the poor.

Give somebody to eat dry corn for a week and you will see him transformed. For naughty children, the mother shall apply the same regime.

If a child is capricious, obstinate, the mother shall give him two nuts. The number two is magnetic method. If the child is unbalanced in nature, give him three nuts or apples. The number three is a law of balance. Sometimes nuts may affect badly the organism (when taken in large amounts), because they contain lots of iodine. So, nuts are also able to poison someone. If you want to develop the child's sense of justice, give it four nuts. You shall give for feelings, in general - five nuts, religious feelings – seven nuts, critical and philosophical mind - seven nuts. Do not give more than nine nuts to your children.

WAY OF LIFE IN ACCORDANCE WITH THE LAWS OF ANIMATE NATURE (PREVENTION)

Carnivorousness and Vegetarianism

Fruits are the original human food. The other types of food - meat, fish - are the result of human interpretations and human morality.

The future of people is determined by the food they consume. The cleaner and more healthy food is, the greater and brighter future they prepare for themselves. Therefore, in order food to be cleaned by the toxins that come from the earth, on the one hand, and on the other hand, from the animals, it must be purified. No physical or chemical means are able to purify food from the psychic poisons, besides thoughts and feelings of people. Meat contains the largest amounts of psychic poisons.

There was a time when the earth was like a paradise, vegetation was so rich. There were thousands and millions of fruits and people ate only fruits, but an ice age came on the Earth due to known physical reasons. Then this fertility of the earth decreased and as a result of that people started to eat meat, to exterminate and eat not only animals, but also each other.

For the lower animals, meat is needed as food, but for a higher life, such as the human one, meat is harmful. It impedes the process of human evolution. The elements in people's blood depend on food. The meat of today's mammals that people eat is unclean. Knowing this, they shall keep the purity of their blood, because health depends on it. The human mental health also depends on it.

Carnivorousness leads to suffering, misfortunes, and diseases. To get rid of them, vegetarian food is recommended. Therefore, vegetarianism is not nothing, but a method of treatment. While being treated, people and nations have to eat leaves, i.e. plant food. Then they will come to the real food – fruit-eating, which was the original human food in paradise. In other words: the true human food includes bright thoughts, lofty feelings, and noble deeds. These are the fruits of life that people have to eat in the future.

Today the question about what type of food to be eaten is raised: meat or vegetarian? Vegetarian food is preferable. Why? One of the scientific explanations, which support vegetarianism, is that the minds of the animals, which are slaughtered, are quite developed. They want to live. They do not go voluntarily to be slaughtered. However, violence is exercised on them. Violence brings into the body of these animals different poisons that go into the human body. Animals anticipate that they will be slaughtered and begin to embarrass. That embarrassment, that fear, that hatred are the reasons for the poisons that occur in their organisms. One day chemists will investigate these poisons and will be convinced of the truth of these statements.

Fear and loathing, felt by that animals while being slaughtered, introduce these poisons into their organisms. By eating meat, people take in these poisons and get upset. This is the reason for people getting ill of neurasthenia.

According to the structure of the human organism, modern people are is not able to draw out more energy from meat than from other foods that are considered to be weak. Why is that? It is because modern people are very greedy and think that the power of food depends on its quantity or its quality, but not on the way it is used.

The meat of animals is not so nourishing, because, during their feeding process, they use for themselves the valuable nutrients and leave the useless ones, and namely those that people use for food.

The food, used by pigs, supports their organisms and what is more is accumulates as meat and fat.

When someone eats pork, he puts these cells to work, he employs workers for his body, but to put a pig cell to work, you shall put three servants to keep it, not run away somewhere.

The costs for keeping it, costs more than the fulfilled work.

Meat food now is not hygienic and does not establish favorable conditions for the human development, because the vibrations of that food are of another type, inapplicable to humans. Since these creatures are less developed, they lead to people's getting down to the ground. Therefore, one, who eats meat, prepares the his conditions for his destruction. There are people, who cannot even eat some vegetable foods. For example, the stomach of many people does not accept beans. Therefore, we have to come to that food that suits the new life.

People of the new sixth race will be fed with vegetable and fruit food. Meat is a strong food, but harmful and will not be mentioned at all in the future. Carnivorousness is one of the reasons for cruelty and rudeness of people and for neurasthenia. Organism will be recreated through food. If one does not accept fruits as main food, he will live with the stimulus of animals for a long time.

All people, who eat meat aim at the center of the earth. This is their movement. Anyone, who aims at the Sun, is a fruit-eater or a vegetarian. These two directions define what your food will be. You cannot be a vegetarian until you change the direction of your movement toward the Sun.

The danger of vegetarianism for some people is in the fact that they have animal stimulus and want to live in a human way. A certain conflict in the stomach occurs with such people and they say that vegetarianism is not good for them. One has to be a vegetarian by conviction. Then he will be able to properly digest the food he eats.

Meat has introduced such poisons in your organism that today it is a unity of impurities. If you had a normal sense of smell, you would stay far from each other – the smell of those, who eat meat, is so bad. When somebody tells me that he is ailing, the first condition for improvement of his health is to change the food he eats. "What shall we eat then?" The answer is - fruits.

What will one gain if he eats? Will he become stronger. However, if he eats vegetable food, he will become cleaner. Carnivorous animals are stronger, more cruel, more predatory. If you are a wolf, you will eat meat. If you are a sheep, you will eat grass. The desires of the wolf are desires of the Black Lodge, and the desires of the sheep are desires of the White Lodge.

Carnivorousness is the disobedience of God's law.

In order to understand which food is healthier, let us do the following experiment: we will put somebody on a diet - three months we will give him to eat only pork and three times a day he will drink half a liter of wine. We will put another on a fruit diet. In the course of two months he will eat exclusively fruits and drink clean hot water. We will watch both of them during the experiment and will see what their relationships with their relatives and people round them will be.

You may eat meat and cheese, but they cannot create in you a clean body, a noble mind.

One, who cannot avoid meat, cannot get rid of evil. Blood is purified through food. A full vegetarian may be the one, whose ancestors, the previous four or five generations, were vegetarians.

Pigs are the most unclean animals, and so is their meat. One thinks that together with his gut disposal all impurities are removed. Wheat is the purest food.

People die, because carnivorousness exists.

I deny meat, because I know that all crimes throughout the world are due only to it. One, who eats meat, will suffer for sure.

The extreme killing of mammals creates an anomaly in Nature. Most diseases are due to that killing, which stops their evolution, and all powers that shall create their welfare remain unused, thus forming a chaotic state, which is the reason for the various diseases. Do you know what happens after the animal blood flows out promiscuously? From the evaporation - various serums and favorable conditions for harmful germs form and from there evils in the organic world come.

No one, who eats pork or goat, may become great. John the Baptist ate honey and locusts. He was very energetic. Honey softened his character. Locusts imparted gaiety and good mood.

You have studied fruit-eating with angels, and you have studied carnivorousness with the fallen spirits. Carnivorousness came into the world when it was broken the connection of the human soul with God, with Love.

Since all pig cells are highly individualized, when they get into our bodies, we need to spend twice more energy to keep them. These cells are very extremely lazy and we need to hire other workers to do their job – do not hire workers from a pig to work for you. You will hire wonderful workers from potatoes, corn, carrots, cabbage, Jerusalem artichoke, pears, cherries, peppers, who work perfectly well even without payment.

If one knows what harmful elements are contained in pork, rabbit and frog meat, would never smell them, nor eat them.

Fish has a particular magnetic power, needed by the human organism. The same magnetic power may be found in plants, even in larger quantity than in fish. In exceptional cases, one may eat fish.

So, hygiene of life must begin with the proper use of light, stored in plants and fruits. If the perceived light cannot be turned into a living energy, we say that the food is not properly assimilated, i.e. there is no conformity between the given organism and the food. Contemporary hygienists and physiologists often recommend people such foods, with which the desired aim cannot be achieved. Some hygienists recommend people meat, and others – vegetarian food, but sometimes vegetarian food of some oils spoils so much that it may upset your stomach even more than meat. In order to avoid these disorders, one must get to that food, which Nature has determined for him. This is one of the important issues, on which each rational person should think. No matter what is written in books on the subject, each person has to find his own food as animals do. With regard to the choice of food, Nature has put an internal instinct in humans or an internal sense of recognition. And if one goes back to his original state of purity, he will come to a position to distinguish which food is a good and determined especially for him.

Never overeat. Do not give your stomach what it wants. Not everything is nice and useful. Only when you are a vegetarian by conviction, food is properly assimilated.

If one eats mainly meat, he roughens. What may replace meat? Beans may replace meat. In order it to be easily digestible, its peels shall be removed. Then it is an excellent food. It is well beans to be consumed at least once a week.

The character and stability of human beliefs are determined by food, which one eats. Many people think that if they eat meat and varied food they will become physically strong, healthy, and stout. First of all, stoutness does not indicate that a person is healthy, and on the other hand, stoutness does not depend only on food. Food is good if it is able to organize the powers of his organism. Each cell must be organized, alive, to take conscious participation in the functions of human organs. If it does not take part, it is dead, harmful to the organism.

According to the food we consume, people are divided into carnivorous ones and vegetarians. There are vegetarians from birth, but there are vegetarians who consume vegetable foods since 10-20 years. When we talk about vegetarians and compare them to carnivorous people, we consider the first category. The head of vegetarians compared to people, who eat meat, is longer and narrower, while the head of the people, who eat meat, is wider and shorter. In general, the head of the carnivorous people is wider around the ears. This indicates that the destructive abilities are highly developed in them. Food affects the physical, spiritual and mental lives of people.

So far, the most clean and hygienic food is the vegetable one. A day will come when the plants in an effort to keep their lives will begin to release poisons that will do harm to people. Today, there are also plants that release substances, which are harmful for the human organism. People use these poisons in limited quantity as medicines.

What is the benefit of being vegetarians and not eating meat, but you have not changed your thoughts and feelings? Not only in form, but in substance, if you do not alter your diet, your thoughts and feelings, you cannot change your life.

A true vegetarian shall use clean food, clean thoughts, feelings and deeds.

By fasting, starvation, one can get rid of the fat, but he cannot gain a gift. Fasting strengthens the will, but gift is not developed in him. Through it one realizes that he will not die of hunger. People have inherited the excessive eating.

Eating corn and fruits is one thing, and eating all sorts of meat is another. For food we shall not cause sufferings to any creature, because this stumbles ourselves.

In the future, people will eat only fruits like angels do.

Vegetable food is not so clean for introducing the elements of immortality.

A day will come when people will not eat meat. A day will come when people will not eat vegetable food too. Then they will eat like angels do - with the pure nectar of Nature.

Do you think that Nature approves the food of contemporary people? It has created fruits and vegetables – food ready to be eaten by humans. But not knowing how to use it, they boil them, fry them, add various spices. But instead of favor that food brings harm to them.

You shall learn to cook from Nature. Just look at the fruits. And you, when you chop the meat and add onion, red and black pepper, various fragrances and spices, and the final result is a mess!

The power of the food that may be used by our stomach, does not depend on how it is cooked. Do not think that if you put a little more salt, pepper and oil, the food will be healthier - it all will be for our taste. In order to test whether a given food is good, we shall what is its effect on our stomach after half an hour. If you feel a little weight, this food does not suit your health.

It is preferable less salt to be added to food, and one, who needs more salt, he himself adds the needed amount. Water is a bearer of life, but not salt.

If you want to benefit of nutritive value of the beans, cook it without spices. Cook it in clean water, with one or two onions, without olive oil. If you add oil, you will spoil it. The bean contains a special oil, which is in disagreement with the other types of oil or with peppers. Seed beans within clean places, exposed to the sun. Never eat beans that have been in cellars for more than one year.

Old Bulgarians threw the first water, in which the beans had boiled, as unhealthy, and they boiled the beans in another water. I would like Bulgarians to return to the old folk traditions that rested on the very important psychological laws and have good results.

Never eat old or not well boiled beans. It is a symbol of human selfishness. It is nourishing. It gives a lot, but it also takes a lot.

Do not add salt while boiling beans.

If you want your food to become good, you may bake a little the onion or boil it, but do not fry it. Onion is healing when eaten raw, baked or boiled.

When frying onion, meat, and other foods, all volatile oils are lost and some of the nourishing substances disappear. You need to know what elements to use in cooking and how to combine them.

One, who wants to be healthy, shall not eat fried onions. Only one, who is ill, may eat fried onion as medicine. One, who wants to be healthy, shall eat food, cooked by someone who loves him.

Wheat and Bread

Wheat grain is a symbol of the human soul. It is a great history in the development of Nature. It has strength, ability, spirit of renunciation, with which it feeds itself and the others. It is a great mystery.

Wheat grain is one of the beloved children of angels. The more you chew it, the more you gain.

Wheat is the purest food.

So far, there is no healthier food than wheat. However, the way wheat is milled and bread prepared, most of its nutritional substances are lost.

A lot from the Sun is incorporated in the wheat grain and if you were able to absorb that valuable content from it, you would not need any other food. All other foods come in addition to wheat and bread.

If we knew how to use food, we would not need any other food, but wheat. By changing your state, you will attract all those elements that are contained in wheat. Let's assume that you want to draw elements for your mind. What do you do? You will harness the nitrogen substances to work, by constantly thinking about the spiritual world, the God of love. Only then you will draw those elements from the wheat, introduced by the Sun and needed for you. If you want to draw energy for your feelings, your heart, you shall harness oxygen to work.

I prefer raw wheat to warm baked bread. There are vitamins in wheat, which disappear during bread baking. During milling of the wheat by millstone, a big part of its nutritional substances are lost.

Milling of wheat is a human invention. There will no be mills in future culture. It is best raw wheat to be eaten, but as modern people do not have healthy teeth, wheat shall be boiled and eaten in this form, while it is still warm. If the cooked wheat stays overnight, it should not be eaten. Fresh wheat shall be boiled every day.

You can eat wheat in its natural from, but you may also bake it as bread. If you take a pear, you may bake it and eat it, but you may also eat it in its natural form. The wheat, the pear, and all fruits have been baked once by the Sun. There is an internal process in Nature, in which life manifests. When the wheat grain grows and matures, it gains life in itself. However, when the wheat grain is baked, it does not gain life.

It is not needed the wheat to be milled. It is enough it to be smashed and eaten in this way.

I think that people shall not eat much. They need little food, which shall be digested. Nothing shall remain in the stomach. Food shall be completely digested. Nothing shall remain. The body burning should also be complete and excessive gases shall not be released. Indeed, if one could take out the entire energy from the wheat, he would be able to sustain his life with the help of only 100 grams of wheat for a week. And how many times do modern people eat per 100 g of wheat in the course of a week? In addition, it is fact that people consume rather little energy from the food they eat!

What should one eat at a physical level? The answer is bread - the most important thing. Eating is a blessing that God has given and its task is great.

Bread contains within itself all nutritional materials. One may perfectly well live only by bread, fruits, and water. It is important people to chew very well and eat with love, gratitude and in good mood. People cripple themselves by in eating whatever they wish and in a hurry, without chewing. They do not know how to eat, how to sleep, how to breathe, and they want to be healthy.

The pure wheat bread has more nutrients than other foods. One may live even if he eats only bread. When kneading bread with yeast, the living ferments multiply and live, releasing useless substances. So Moses forbade Jews to knead leavened bread.

Bread should be made of new, fresh wheat to be healthy.

It is preferable bread to be baked well to remaining underbaked.

Bread is given to people by grace and as a blessing. If your teeth are healthy, eat raw wheat grains. There is no need of milling and baking it.

Bread is the most necessary and sacred food for humans. It does not bring these profits, because it is prepared with insults, quarrels and discontent.

From all foods, wheat and bread are the best. All other foods come to supplement the bread.

Fasting

Hunger is a power in the world that still lives. Not suffering, but hunger prolongs life, makes it more intense.

One of the conditions for prolonging life is hunger. One, who wants to achieve something great, must hunger, eat less.

One, who may hunger and knows how to hunger, prolongs his life. All good, rational, and great people were hungering.

To be healthy and strong, one shall voluntarily hunger from time to time. Hunger strengthens the organism. It makes sense one to hunger, but not overhunger. Nature uses hunger as a great, powerful engine. All chemical reactions are based on hunger. The aim of the elements to be satisfied is not nothing else, but satisfaction of their hunger. Conscious hunger prolongs life.

True fasting is a method of regulation of the feelings and thoughts of people. Fasting is not only not eating and drinking and not eating of fats and meat, but during fasting one shall take in sublime thoughts and feelings, to be ready to reconcile with all his enemies and pay all his debts.

If you want to perform all of your obligations, to remove all misfortunes, fast for 5-10-15-20 days, but only if your heart and mind suggest that. In a certain moment of life, when we must strengthen our will and unite it with the will of God, we must fast.

If you feel any abnormal condition of you organism, spend one or two days in fasting, drink more hot water, breathe air and be in light.

Before starting to fast, you should take a purgative to clean your stomach well. It makes sense one to fast man, but only if he can clean his thoughts and feelings. If he does not achieve that, fasting is useless. On the other hand, fasting is needed for a rest of the organism – internal and external. Fasting is recommended as a means of healing. In times of fasting, burning in organism is more intense, as a result of which all substances that cause various diseases, ailments and dissatisfactions are burned.

What does fasting mean at a physical level? Its goal is not you to become feeble, yellow, and weak, but not to torture your husband, wife, and neighbor. Not to make him wear torn or dirty socks or shoes, or clothes. You shall do so: you will sew or knit clothes, socks for him, or you will buy him something new and nice. The shoes are to be nice and comfortable. Do not make him sleep on a ragged straw-mattress, do not suspect him that he deals with somebody else's women. Consider him as a saint. This is fasting.

On Fridays you shall not cook and eat cooked food. You may eat only bread with a few olives or bread with some fruits. You may choose one of the Fridays of the month, during which you will eat nothing. If something happens and one cannot fast on the relevant Friday, then next month he will fast during two Fridays. You shall tell nobody when you are going to fast, or when you fast, or when you have fasted. Some of you, who may, let them fast for 40 hours, but at least 24 complete hours. Everybody shall fast. One day per a month is not much at all. How many Fridays during the year does it make?

You shall devote the whole ninth day of the month to God. You will eat fruits during that day.

If breathe consciously during a hunger, you may take enough nourishing energy from the air. One may eat himself fill even only with Love. That Love will first pass through the air, and the air is able to do everything in humans and give a right thought. This right thought you will project to someone, who has hungered for a few days, and he will be sated.

One, who goes on an excursion, shall not fast. He shall carry bread, drink water and thank God. On an excursion everyone shall be sated. The main idea of fasting is the hidden in the cells energy to be awaken and the organism to be renovated. If you fast without a reason, it is useless. In addition, the relevant periods for fasting shall be obeyed. If you start on

Monday, you will have one result, on Tuesday - another, etc. And if you start it at noon, in the morning, or in the evening, you will have different results. If certain rules are not obeyed, you will have no successful attempts. The Bible says that Elijah fasted 40 days to magnetize. Fasting is a tool for removing fear, to control the blood circulation and brain. People shall be always alert, because then he becomes very sensitive, attracts dynamic natural powers and needs to know how to deal with them.

Not only the physical fasting and hunger treat, but also the spiritual one. While fasting, you will breathe more. By fasting you strengthen your will and thus you endure more work, learning, thinking.

It is well one to satisfy his desire, but it is better if he educates it. Many people fast, torture their bodies, without understanding the meaning of the fasting. One should fast consciously. When he notices a negative feature in himself, a negative thought or feeling, he may fast for two or three days to get rid of that negative thing.

In my opinion 24 hours of conscious fasting is equivalent to 10 days of mechanical fasting. Within 24 hours of conscious fasting, one may renovate the cells of his body. Fast 24 hours and be merry and joyful. Sing and thank God for everything. When 24 hours pass, feed and thank again for the bread, water. The number 24 is harmonious. It is related to the rotation of the Earth around its axis. It will put you in harmony with the Earth.

Fasting is not for torturing your body, but a diet for harmonizing mental powers; for regulating the flows in you and apply them. The extreme fasting, the extreme abstinence created the opposite process - gluttony.

Breathing

Breathing is the first condition that gives people certain virtues. When one learns to breathe properly, he must proceed to proper nutrition.

As long as there is air, there is mental life too. The air is connected to the mind. Within the physical world, people breathe through the lungs. There are people, who have also achieved internal breathing - through the astral and mental bodies.

The materials, which the brain uses, are of higher, fine matter. You cannot change your breathing if you do not change your mind and vice versa. Breathing is the first condition that gives people certain virtues. Breathing is a measure for determining the level of human development. One, who breathes properly, can modify the state of his digestive and respiratory systems and be a master of the lower powers in himself. If one cannot manage his stomach, he cannot regulate the powers related to it. The Scriptures says: "and breathed into his nostrils the breath of life; and man became a living soul." So, God introduced the soul of man through his nose and made from him a living soul. Figuratively, his soul is in his chest, in the respiratory system. That is why we say that the solar plexus is the seat of his soul. Proper breathing does not depend on the quantity of the inhaled air, but on the duration of its holding. If one wants to know how much his power is, let him check by a clock for how long he holds the breath. Some adepts have come to a level of holding it for half an hour or for one hour. The longer you can hold it, the farther you can go for a walk outside the Earth. It will come a day when man will not only breathe through his lungs, but through the whole body. All cells will take in air from outside, will keep dirt inside them, and direct completely clean air toward the lungs. There will not be unachievable things for him.

When the spring is setting in, start to go for a walk every morning. The earlier you go out, the better. Breathe deeply. First clean the machine, adjust, and then start working. If you do not do this in advance, it will surprise you at a moment, at which you do not expect. And then instead of one hour, you will spend ten hours until putting it in good working order. Full breathing means breathing not only by the lungs, but also by the skin of the whole body. Each cell shall breathe. The organism does not tolerate any impurities, no alien substances. If such things gather, one gets ill. Each disease starts releasing the organism from these substances. If any of the small channels of the spine gets blocked, one loses his vitality. The spinal cord has the ability to absorb food from the air and transmit it to the whole organism.

One major and important issue in life is breathing. However, you breathe through your skin too - seven million pores participate in breathing and if they get blocked, one dies. If you do not breathe through both the lungs and the skin, you are exposed to various diseases. While breathing, keep your head upright, exactly perpendicular to the ground.

If one entangles his physical works, i.e. the material ones, his stomach gets upset. It is noticed that some individuals may be physically healthy, without being strong. From where does human power come? It comes from the lungs. If you do not breathe properly, you cannot be strong. The stomach takes an active part in the building of the body. The stomach system manages the physical man; the sympathetic nervous system, connected to the rear portion of the brain, manages the spiritual man; and the nervous system, connected to the cerebrum and the spinal, cord, manages the mental or Divine life of man. In order one to be spiritual, he must understand the functions of the solar plexus. To be strong, he must develop the respiratory system - the lungs. The stomach performs transverse and longitudinal movements, and the lungs - in width. So, food causes one kind of movements in the stomach, and the air in the lungs - another. One has to eat only when he is hungry. By eating properly, you also breathe properly. If you breathe properly, you think properly. The process of thinking will be the same as the process of eating.

There is an element of immortality in the air. Actually this element comes from the Sun. People have knowledge, study and cannot derive the elixir. It passes through them and does not remain in them. In spite of the many breathing systems, Hindus have not touched to that secret of Nature, either.

All people breathe air, but do not perceive it in the same way, and the results are different. Most people breathe with the top of their lungs. We call this shallow breathing. To be healthy, you have to breathe deeply, to take in air through your entire lungs. The deeper breathing is, the greater quantity of energy enters into the lungs, which, together with the air, covers all lung cells and helps for the good cleaning of the blood.

Everything depends on the proper breathing, and it implies to get out all the energy, contained in the air.

When a person does not take enough food from the air, he always feels weak, overworked, without life and powers in himself.

When you breathe, think about Love. When you exhale, think about God's Love. The spine has three channels. Two channels are open – up in the big brain and in the sympathetic nervous system. People breathe through them. The third one – the channel of Truth is closed in modern humans - all evil is there. If this channel, which is in the middle, opens, the air will freely enter the brain. The other two flows will pass from there too. They will go to the front part of the forehead and to the top of the head. Then one will gain the cosmic consciousness, gain a completely different appearance, a completely different power. Since, for now, only the two channels are open, and the most important one is blocked, humans, although great in many respects, are pathetic and helpless. One of the channels in women is more developed, and the other - in men. Children will develop the third channel. The new that is born are our children. All lofty thoughts that come in us are our children.

There are many methods of breathing. They are all nice, but they lack one essential element - intentional breathing. Hindus, for thousands of years, have dealt with breathing as science. They have established entire schools for that and they have achievements in that respect, but no matter how good their methods are, they are not for the Europeans. Europeans do not have these internal states, that spirituality, experiences, depth, attitude to God as Hindus. All this is important in order breathing to be proper and full.

I will give you a breathing method: take a breath and hold it for about 20 seconds and say during that time: "God, for the great good that You give me, I am ready to do Your will." These words come out through the air, go in the space and chronicle. And what you have taken from the air, adapts very well in the organism. And the beings from the other world, listening to you, will perceive that formula, which is a good for them. They will get the good out from the air together with you. You will not say these words only once, but always when you do breathing exercises during the day. By breathing, accompanied by formulas, you can get rid of all oppressive states.

You can get everything you need from the air, if you know how. There is calcium, oil, and what not in the air.

You cannot breathe well and properly, if the mind is not active and clean. Clean mind attracts clean air.

It is worth devoting a lifetime to learn breathing properly. Diseases, sufferings, failures are due to improper breathing. One, who breathes properly, thinks properly. When one thinks properly, his works always arrange well.

As students, you have to pay attention to your breathing. One, who breathes properly, will sing properly. By singing well, you connect to Nature and draw life from it. By singing, one develops inside him, those organs, through which he takes from the air the necessary stamina. And by speaking, one also takes vital energy from the air. Singing and speaking are related to the mind.

Long life depends on the right thinking and feeling, on the deep and proper breathing. Proper breathing helps for forming the character, strengthens the light of the mind, and makes the face beautiful. Wrinkling of the face and hands is due to improper breathing and disorder of the liver.

Each inhalation aims at regulation and cleaning of wishes, and each exhalation is associated with the cleaning of the mind. Clean blood is a prerequisite for a healthy body, and the healthy body - for the proper distribution of the energies in the human organism. The lungs are a sieve, through which the mental and heart lives of man get clean.

You will remember: when you breathe, normally you will do 10-12 inhalations per minute. When you practice, you will take 4 to 1 breaths per minute. You will start with 4 and will gradually go down. If you get to one inhalation and one exhalation per minute, you have acquired many.

If a person wants to be healthy, he shall get to 10 inhalations per minute. If they increase to 20 inhalations per minute, you will pay a high price. This is already not life.

There is a link between poor memory and breathing. At weak, improper breathing, too little prana enters the brain.

Concentration of the mind and memory strengthening depend mainly on deep breathing. One should love, in order the future respiratory organs for taking in the ether to develop in him. Love organizes the ether doppelganger of man.

For development of patience, I especially recommend you to breathe deeply. Patience is related to breathing, to the respiratory system. The deeper one breaths, the more patient he is. Breathe deeply and hold your breath for 10 – 20 - 30 or more seconds. Patience increases in a ratio to the seconds. If a person breathes properly, deeply, for 1 - 2 years, he will develop in himself a certain gift and abilities. He will become more patient, more thoughtful, will develop his imagination, and will gain more calmness.

One, who breathes rapidly, he has a weak will. Apply your will while breathing and gradually reduce the number of inhalations: from 20 go down to 19, 18, 17, 16, 15. If you can get to 10 inhalations per minute, this will have a healthy effect on your organism.

One, who wants to strengthen his will, has to breathe slowly.

One must begin to hold air in his lungs from 20 seconds and increase by a few seconds every day. If he achieves this, he can easily cope with difficulties and contradictions.

The average person inhales 20 times and exhales 20 times per minute. Talented people inhale and exhale by 10 times per minute. The genius inhales and exhales by 4 times per minute. The saint inhales and exhales by one time per minute.

Water

Warm water is the elixir of the new life.

To be healthy, one must drink a certain amount of water, which, on one hand, is needed for softening the food, and on the other hand - for washing the internal organs. No reaction can take place without water.

Water contains a vital power needed for the human body, and syrups, no matter how nice they are, are invented by humans. They cannot quench thirst.

If you know how to drink boiling water, it will bring into you such elements that 90% of the modern crises, which corrode the society, will disappear.

Drinking and washing by water for you shall be a sacred act. You shall wash slowly, intently. You shall drink water with a focused mind and by saying formulas. Find where the best water is. You shall bring water from the cleanest springs.

If you drink cold water, your mind should be awake. Many diseases are generated by the rapid drinking of cold water. When one drinks cold water, he must think, his mind should take full part in the sweetness of water and its temperature. If you hurry when you drink water, you will lose more time to heal from the consequences than if you have used one or two minutes for drinking up water.

After something warm never drink something cold, because teeth decay as a result of the rapid temperature changes. Nature does not like sudden changes, and what good will the expansion and contraction of the tooth enamel bring?

You shall drink water, on an empty stomach, from 100 to 150 grams, in

213

swallows. You shall drink per half a liter - one liter of water a day, from which you will be able to take out food for your arteries.

Never drink cold, icy water to prevent excessive contraction of the capillaries in the throat and in the stomach. Never breathe through the mouth, but through the nose in order the air to be cleaned and warmed due to the slimy membrane and fluid in the nose.

To bathe is not a pleasure, but a necessity, imposed by the need of the body to open the pores of the skin, through which breathing and eating happen normally. Moreover, one shall remain in water from 5 to 15 minutes, no more.

Water, containing organic impurities, has a harmful effect on the body. Distilled water improves health. Each day one should drink at least a liter or a liter and a half of water.

Cold compresses and showers are for powerful people, the circulation of whom is normal. Someone takes a hot shower, and then enters a cold pool. After that he wonders why his state has deteriorated. Rapid temperature changes do not have a good effect on the organism.

Someone says: I take cold showers to toughen. Until one toughens, these drastic changes will cause various effects of hardening of the body, due to which more electricity will accumulate in the organism, with which he will hardly cope.

As for the cold baths, I would recommend to everyone rainy baths, mainly during the months of May, June, July till the middle of August at the latest. The rainy drops during these months are warm and full of electricity and magnetism. Rainy baths in the remaining months are not recommended.

When you cannot take rainy baths, it is better to take baths with water that is heated to a maximum of 35 - 40°C - close to the natural body temperature. Such are many of the natural springs. Above this temperature, water has already a tensile strength that is not pleasant for the body.

It is good rainy baths not to be taken straight on the body, but through a thin article of clothing. Taken in this way, the baths, the raindrops develop a special energy that affects the body favorably.

Part of the water is taken in through the skin pores. So one has to wash his face frequently and then water penetrates into the pores and part of the magnetism of the water penetrates into the skin with it. Water should be warm in order this to happen. There is a connection between the physical purity and the spiritual one.

One must at least twice a week induce sweating by drinking hot water. He will drink a few glasses of hot water, in which he can squeeze a few drops of lemon juice. When he sweats well, he will wipe his body with a damp towel and will change his clothes. Then let him drink another half or a whole cup of hot water. The clean hot water helps for releasing blood from the accumulated in it lactic and uric acid. To be healthy, one must have absolutely clean blood. Once a person improves his circulation, prana is taken in properly by the body.

In order your breathing to be full, you should open the pores of your body. This is achieved through drinking of water. Full breathing means one to breathe not only through his lungs, but also through the skin of his body. Every cell in the human body shall breathe. One, who breathes in this way, can be called a healthy person.

Hands, at least three times a day, shall be washed. Legs, face, underarms shall be washed several times a day, leaving the skin slightly damp in order the remaining water to be taken in by the body and give you liveliness and freshness. Wipe, lightly, with a soft towel. Then change your clothes and thank God and after all that, you may eat or go to work.

In summer, warm the water in the sun and wash yourself by solar water. You shall take two or three baths a week. You can wash yourself partially every day and namely the face, the neck, the arms, the legs. When you perspire, you shall immediately change your clothes.

Never drink water when you are tired and sweating. Stop for a while at the spring, wait for 10 - 15 minutes and then drink.

If wine were a necessity for people, Nature should deliver it. Water cleans the body, and wine introduces sludge, from which one must clean himself in order the Divine energy to enter it. This energy comes in through the brain, through the heart and through the body. Once this energy enters the human body, it starts to rebuild it.

Dew drops have electricity and magnetism, which must be used wisely. Knowing this, do not shake the raindrops out of your clothes. The clean dew drop gives blessing. One, who has a strong sense of smell, feels the fragrance of the dew drops.

When you go for a walk or hike, choose to drink water that has southern exposure, because spring water, placed in such a position is full of creative energy and they are healthy. Never drink water exposed to the north, because their energy is positive.

From May till the middle of July, every day, when it rains, you shall stay out under the rain until you get wet well. Officials will use those hours when they are not at work. These rain baths cost more than mineral ones, and they are beneficial to the nervous system and to many chronic diseases. I call rain baths "baths of angels". While taking your baths, you will pray to God to clean you through them and thank for the blessing that He sends you from Heaven. One, who can correctly take in the energies of the raindrops, has reached that primary matter, which alchemists sought. By taking these baths, you will see how well you will sleep. After the bath, you will wipe your body with a clean, dry towel. You will change your clothes, and drink a glass or two of hot water. As for the cold, you shall not have any fear. May, June, and July are full of life.

Sun

People shall get up early in the morning, go out in fresh air, and meet the first sun rays that contain a specific energy for all living organisms. No matter for how long one suns himself at noon, he will gain nothing.

Expose your back to the sun, connect with its energy when you feel well, as well as when you do not feel well and observe the results. You shall know during which hours of the day to do that in order to take in only its beneficial rays. There are rays, which tire you. If one is a farmer, he is to wear a hat in the form of a polygon to refract the sun's harmful rays.

Never stand in the shadow of a tree or in the shadow of somebody else. This is a rule that everybody may try. Each ray, which has fallen on you, is absorbed by your organism and then comes out again in the form of light, called dead light. There is light in the shadow of a flower, of a tree, or in the shadow of a house, but it is called dead light. Therefore, you have to be under the influence of the direct sun rays, but not under the indirect ones, i. e. the shadow rays. Never stand in a shadow. These rules can be summarized, be tried and become knowledge.

Thoughts

Thoughts and feelings determine your state in the world: what friends you will have, what status you will have, and your health – everything depends on the mind.

One's thoughts and behavior determine his destiny and his status in life. His mind and his behavior determine his place in life – whether he will be rich or poor, healthy or sick, happy or unhappy.

If you do not think properly, you cannot be healthy.

Through the thought man collects three types of energy, of which he builds his mental body, which he takes with him to the other world. Immortality is the mental body of man.

The human power is in the thought. The thought, like bread, feeds people. If your thoughts are not healthy, no matter how much you eat, you will languish. One, who lives by the laws of love, faith and hope, may be healthy and joyful even if he eats only dry pieces of bread. The Word of God is the living bread, about which Christ spoke. It is a compressed Divine energy.

What one constantly thinks will come and what he constantly denies will also come. If you think that you will get rich, you will get rich. If you think that you will get into trouble, you will get into trouble. If you think that you will fall ill, the disease will come.

Man does not create thoughts. He only takes them in and delivers them. Thoughts that pass through the human mind come from rational beings in the mental world. Their thoughts fill the whole space. Everyone takes in such thoughts that vibrate equally with his mental apparatus.

Do not think that someone can create a thought by himself. You shall attract the harmonic thought from creatures that are much higher than you. The same applies to feelings. The Divine thought is transmitted by the light, by the air, by the soil, by plants, stones. One, who understands the laws, can draw from everywhere.

Like thoughts you have, like creatures you contact.

A bright and lofty thought, repeated often, sincerely, and unselfishly, delivers something to a person. Nature rewards for every good word, for every good thought, addressed to someone. In this way, one may help himself at various diseases. A healthy person often thinks of a disease and attracts it. Do exactly the opposite - think of health to attract and strengthen it. The rational, good, great in man is able to fight microbes that cause diseases.

There is no organ in the human body, which is not governed by some kind of thoughts and feelings. By knowing this, keep your mind and heart in good order, in order they to be able to perceive properly the thoughts and feelings that come from the higher world.

In order your brain to be in good state, keep away from contradictory thoughts. In order the solar plexus to be in good state, never allow negative feelings in your heart.

There are thoughts in people, which are highly electrical, thus causing large explosions in the nervous system. These explosions gradually destroy the human organism. Beware of thoughts that destroy the nervous system.

Mind creates miracles. The large stones of the pyramids were lifted and moved by a strong mind.

You can help thousands of people through your mind.

There are circular links in the mind. A thought may have passed through a chain of 10 - 20 000 people until it is implemented by somebody.

Each right thought that passes through your mind, after passing through the minds of all people, and even through the whole heaven, will return to you. And if it was right, will bring the entire wealth with itself. If it was wrong, it will return with all weaknesses, which it has, and of course, you will feel its load.

Each projected thought comes out as a stream and moves wave-like through the space. When the human thought is intense, it creates vary beautiful forms. By the form of these waves you can guess about what your friend thinks.

Every thought produces a particular color.

The wrong thought affects blood circulation and therefore the activity of all organs.

A person with a strong mind can go to patients with plague, or cholera and come out unharmed. One may get ill from fear without any germs.

If one allows negative thoughts in his mind, an aura of negative and opposing thoughts and powers will form round him. Then severe conditions will occur, and this is an accumulation of excess energy that is not natural, and a way shall be found for its transformation. This energy is not Divine. You shall immediately oppose Divine, bright, clean thoughts to the negative ones.

There are certain words that produce cold waves, and there are other words that produce warmth in people, and others - light. There are words that produce darkness in us.

In order to be healthy, keep in good state the brain and the sympathetic nervous system. When the brain is in a harmonious state, it can cure all diseases. If one negative thought comes into it, ailments, diseases, disorders immediately appear. This is one of the reasons for memory fading and mind confusion.

When one thinks improperly, blood rushes into the cerebellum, where passions and ordinary feelings are. Sexual activity awakens and he gives in to unnatural feelings. Lower feelings contribute nothing. This is spiritual drunkenness. Human, personal love leads to drunkenness.

When our thought is unclean, carbon dioxide increases. When our clean thought increases, oxygen also increases, and carbon decreases. When the heart is clean, oxygen increases.

Once you start thinking badly, you suffocate, breathing is not normal.

As long as one's consciousness is awake, no illness is able to attack him. A disease, cold, alien substances do not enter his organism.

Beware of your bad thoughts and feelings, as well as of those of the others round you.

It is a law: good life makes blood clean. The moment, at which a person brings an unclean thought in his mind and an unclean feeling in his heart, the blood loses its purity. Each bite, which is not accompanied by a good thought, brings poison to the stomach.

Each negative thought attracts to itself the relevant poisonous substances, which introduces a certain dissonance both in man himself and in Nature.

How will you cope with your negative, gloomy conditions? Sit quietly at one place for 5 - 10 minutes, relax your muscles, there shall be no pressure, and start thinking about good and beautiful things. Imagine beautiful pictures, images until you come in good mood.

One bad and one good thought can balance their energies. Therefore, if a negative thought enters your mind, do not strive for throwing it out, but immediately oppose to it a good thought. If you use violence or something bad against it, it will double its energies and will cause greater mischief. Answer by good to the bad and evil. This is implied in the verse, said by Christ: "Resist not evil".

Vary your thoughts. There is nothing worse than the uniform thought. It is like a hammer hitting at a single place.

Catching a cold depends on the human mind. There are people, who live and work with open windows for years and do not catch a cold.

Therefore if monotony appears in your life and the effect of this is sedative, start taking such thoughts into your head, which to bring some variety. It is better if you alone take them into your head and influence yourself than if others influence you. One can make use of suggestion to strengthen his health, to develop his abilities, to strengthen his memory, etc. In whatever conditions you are, keep in your mind a positive thought that you can still find a fertile soil to work.

Each bad thought is a dissonance. Correct it immediately. Dissonance is two scales that are disharmonious. There is no correspondence between them. Replace immediately the bad thought by a bright and harmonious one.

Glands are to be developed. When you are in a difficulty, turn your attention to the gland, which is in the throat, or to the one that is in the pit of the stomach and you will get a response on how to get out of the difficulty.

Think for two minutes on the words "love" and "agreement". If you do it for ten minutes a day, you will see the results. You shall strive to have harmony in your mind at each moment. Your mind should get used to focusing. It diverts a lot, but when you focus on harmony for 1-2 minutes, your mind will get used to focusing. By doing exercises, your cells, your nerves will start to train and if you have a headache or any discomfort, it will pass. If you do exercises of the kind, you can be treated. Each treatment is cleaning, and cleaning is health. By doing exercises for harmony, everything in you will be cleaned.

Air, water, fire, and earth – these four elements are symbols and show the different types of matter, of which man is made. There is consciousness and life in these elements. If a person attracts a certain type of matter through his thoughts, he will also acquire states and moods relevant to the matter. If he attracts solid matter by his thoughts, some hardening will also take place in him. People are worried what will happen to them when they get older, who will look after them and in this way they attract solid matter toward them and begin to harden and suffer with atherosclerosis. The latter disease occurs, because of disbelief. To make an old man to turn to God means your hair to turn white.

While thinking, you will often notice light, bright dots that appear from the left and then go the right and disappear. When the dots go from left to right, the thought that is projected towards you, is ascending. That thought is useful. And when that light dot goes from right to left, it is descending. This idea is dangerous and useless for you.

To be healthy, you have to connect mentally with good, strong, healthy people who have no weaknesses and infirmities and take a part of their energy. If you want to get up early, grab the thumb of your left hand with the thumb and forefinger of your right hand and say: "I want to get up tomorrow at 4 a.m." Do the same with your right hand and say the same words. In this way you connect with the powers of the rational world and call them as witnesses.

Some people have used methods for focusing the mind, however, these methods have bad consequences. Why? Due to this you stop your thoughts, but without knowing how to perceive this energy and how to resend it to the body, blockage occurs in you. You concentrate, block your feelings, stop that accumulated energy and become eccentric. Nature does not like you stopping it. That is why, if you feel a burst of energy, go out in the open air, and play and jump there.

When thoughts are highly concentrated, you will not catch a cold. Never allow in yourself the thought that you may catch a cold. If you allow that thought, you have already invited the disease as a guest.

In order not to catch a chill, one must fence himself. This is achieved in two ways: by concentrating of the mind and through a prayer.

There is not a better fence than the mind.

If you think ill of a good man, there is big danger for you. Never think ill of good people. Bulgarians, due to their ill thoughts of Bogomils, were under slavery for 500 years. And the Jews, due to their bad thoughts of Christ, cannot find peace for two thousand years. Once you start thinking something bad of a good person, change your thought immediately.

Bad people are those, whom God have sent to take the dirt and throw it out. You should respect them, because with the help of their cars, they carry your waste and throw it out. You say that this guy is stinking. His position is such. Always think of those, who bear goodness in themselves. You shall be also grateful for bad people, who take out impurities. You shall thank for all that happens around you.

The new man will talk to atoms and molecules of his body as if they are friends. In the morning, when he gets up, he will ask them how they feel, and if they have an excess of energy in their empty spaces in order to take measures for opening of all paths for this energy to come out. He will make something good and he will liberate them from the excessive load in order to avoid explosion.

If you do not allow any negative thought in your mind for three months, you can rejuvenate. When new energy is introduced into the body, it renovates. The renovation is not mechanical. It is related to the spiritual nature of people.

When human sensitivity increases, the heart line prolongs. An excess of energy accumulates in you, which gathers in the back part of your brain and creates great anxieties and disturbances. To cope with this energy, you should think, and direct it to the front of the brain. If the line of the mind prolongs at the expense of the one of the heart, sensitivity decreases and one gradually loses his warmth and humidity, hardens and gets atherosclerosis. For this reason young people suffer with great sensitivity, which leads them directly to softening in feelings, and old people suffer with dryness, hardening and atherosclerosis. Between feelings and thoughts, between mind and heart, there shall be balance.

If the line of the mind is shorter than the line of heart, you shall attempt, through your mind, to prolong it with at least one millimeter. For that goal, you shall deal with mathematics, physics, metaphysics, philosophy to establish a balance between the powers of the mind and the powers of the heart.

Music

Music is a power. You can achieve everything with the help of music in feelings, thoughts and deeds. Where the mind, heart and will take place, music occurs as a powerful force.

Nothing may be achieved without music. In future, music shall be established as a strictly scientific method during the education of children. That is why it is said in the Bible: "Sing and praise God in your hearts!". You cannot think right if you do not sing and play. You cannot feel right, if you do not sing and play. To be a musician or not, that is another question, but inside you you shall have a well developed sense of music. Musicians bear in themselves a magic wand, a magic power, with which they can do a lot.

Thanks to music one may complete something with the least costs, in the easiest way and with the best results.

Music is the best conductor of God's powers.

Music, as an art of angels, is a connecting unit between the angelic and human worlds.

Music is a time in life and through it you may model all organs of yours. You may model the eyebrows, nose, mouth, ears, hairs, and the stomach to how and how much food to eat. You may also make your life healthy and pleasant.

Man shall be a musical being from head to toe. Arms, legs, eyes, everything shall become musical. Everything shall vibrate in a musical state.

Each harmonious thought is well accepted by the cells. It shall be spoken in a musical way to the body. Neither health, nor growth may happen without music. Heart does not beat in the right way without music, nor may the mind be harmoniously created without music.

Certain deposits of poisons are left by the contemporary life and the quick changes, through which you pass – from a joyful mood to a mournful one. That is why music is used as a means against these poisons.

When music conquers the world, there will not be diseases; even if there are diseases, you will get rid of them easier. When you sing, God's world opens and you take in God's life. If you do not sing, you lose. No matter what happens to you, sing.

One shall sing. These classical songs, these mantras, which the Hindus have, the European psalms, they all are a connection for passing from one world into another – the physical, spiritual and mental worlds.

Music influences well the digestion. Try and you will be convinced.

Sing to be healthy. Good health is known by the desire of somebody to sing.

The major scale is the mind, and the minor scale is the heart, and the harmonious one – the will.

Man is musically made. And now you have to go back to that music, by which you are made. God puts all notes at their right place in the human body. One shall start thinking, feeling, singing in the way God has made him in order to hear the song of the flowers– fragrance is their singing. To hear the song of the stars, of the whole world. Now he gets only the static, defined music, but from the point of view of contemporary music, flowers, water, stars, and angels do not sing. Now our ears are also not adapted to another type of music, but you will listen to that music in future.

While one has music in himself, he thinks right, because each right thought, each right feeling is a correct combination of tones.

There is music with not stave, but with six lines. Six cardinal lines and other subsidiary ones.

I talk a lot about music, but you say: "We are old, singing is for the young people." What is the song of the young people and what is the song of the old ones? Young people sing: "I got up.", and the old ones sing: "I became bent", which means that they have become curvilinear with one more center, with a new center. One, who thinks in a musical way, bends his head, because it is heavy for him. He thinks: this is not arranged, that is not arranged; it hurts him here and there. If he sings to the ill place, because the thought is concentrated in that direction, more blood will come and soon he will recover. Without singing, the capillaries get narrower and the blood circulation does not happen in the right way.

People, who have tender feelings, have music. They may sing and play and stand high in respect to consciousness.

Tones are connected to the planets, to all heavenly bodies. The whole world is a musical composition. All planets have a special tone. All numberless worlds sing at various scales. Supreme beings and all higher hierarchies sing. You cannot be happy without music. You cannot understand Christianity without music. The first songs of the Christians were ordinary and sad, because they were chased and music was not so available. There are creatures in Nature, who does not allow singing. Bulgarians also think that it is not appropriate for an old man to sing.

All old mantras, from the hoary antiquity, are implemented in the songs, which I have given to you. If you sing them in the right way, you will benefit of them. These songs are created in accordance with laws of the future music. These are songs, which do not die. Do you think that they are being created today?

Sing a song to God. If you have made mistakes in singing, do not embarrass. When the song passes through the angles, they will correct it and when it reaches God, He corrects is so that it becomes the best symphony and then he returns it. When a brother or a sister comes and asks you to sing something, sing right away one song, two songs, as many as he wants. Never say that you will spoil your voice in this way. There shall be readiness in music, generosity. If you sing, you will gain. One, who sings, always gains. There is not a singer, who have sung and failed in the angels of music, but all that do not sing, have failed.

All tones are living beings in the Invisible world. "Do" is a specific tone only of certain rational beings. "Re" is a tone of other beings, etc. When we sing the scale, we are in connection to those beings. As long as we sing, they come and we exchange with them. The mind and the heart are the base of the laws of singing. We all, by working together, will achieve what God wants. Many creatures, by singing, by thinking, the thought goes rightly. It is a very hard work for a man to think by himself. While singing, think that you are being helped by the genes of music. The contemporary world may get rid of the sorrows only in this way. When people start singing, they will stop thinking ill.

Sleep

In order to be healthy, one shall know when to go to bed and when to get up. When you go to bed on time, your body will rest, and your spirit will study.

The sleep is the physioastral life on the Earth. Eating is just the physical life on the Earth.

Work is the mental life on the Earth. Only while sleeping, one gains his energies. Eating is a process, during which energies are put into action, and the work is usage of the already gained energies.

A day will come, when people may live without sleep. Sleep is a rest only for those, on whom the rational beings work. In this way their consciousness will raise. In order to come to a higher consciousness, one shall adopt balance between the mind and the heart. When he comes to that balance, the processes in his organism will happen normally.

Sleeping has become necessary for people because of a breach of God's laws. The sleep and death are not foreseen.

The earliest one goes to bed, the better it is for him. Why? Those, who go to bed early, they take in the whole gathered prana, i.e. the vital energy in the atmosphere. Those, who go to bed late, they hardly fall asleep, because there is no enough quantity of prana for their organism. Do not go bed later than midnight. In general, 8 p.m., 10 p.m. and midnight are the hours determined for going to bed.

Contemporary people attract lots of misfortunes, because of lots of sleeping. They do not go to bed on time, when they have to sleep, and they do not get up on time, when they have to get up. Do you know why you cannot sleep? This is very simple. At what time do hens go to bed? They know that when the Sun goes down, there are lots of trains to the other world. The messages for the other world are very good, but later than 10 p.m., 11p.m., and midnight, the trains come more rarely and they will have to wait. You cannot go to the other world. You will be awake at the station, you will wait, but when you get on the train that has arrived, it is easy. It will bring you to the other world.

Contemporary people must go to bed in the evening at 10 p.m. at the latest and get up at 5 a.m. in the morning. One, who wants to live healthfully, he shall go to bed and get up early.

Evil grows mechanically, and good grows organically. Never leave a bad thought to work in your consciousness.

In the evening, before going to bed, review your thoughts and do not leave in your consciousness any bad thought to work, because that bad thought will stop your progress and will do harm to the others, too.

Before going to bed, you shall undress and say to yourselves: "God, thank You for the life and for everything that You gave me. Thank You for the eyes, arms, legs, ears, mouth, heart, for everything that You gave me." You shall thank for everything. You shall touch each part of your body and then go to bed. You shall thank for the mouth and tongue, through which you say sweet words. You have a nice brain. Thank for it. You have ears for hearing, and eyes for looking. Thank for everything.

If you do not know how to sleep, you will never be able to study spiritually. To sleep means to put your body in such a position that, when your doppelganger comes out, to find your teacher, who will teach you, because knowledge is taught in the upper world, the spiritual one, and not on the Earth. When you go to bed, you shall fall asleep in 5-10 minutes. Sleeping is art – you shall get up in the same way (e.g. on the right side), in which you have fallen asleep. The correct way of sleeping will improve your heart.

When you sleep, you go to school in the astral world. What you study in the evening, you apply it during the day. That is why, when you go to bed in the evening, say: "Now I got to the school of the astral world and wish to do a good job, which will be assigned to me there."

Sleeping is a process, during which consciousness shall go out from the organism for it to renovate. If the consciousness does not separate, man cannot rest. Sleeping is a rest, renovation, cleaning. When the consciousness goes out, workers come to clean the body. When one comes back, he sees his body cleaned, ready for work. You shall come out and leave your servants in the body fulfill their work. Man comes in the body and goes out and others work for him. He even does not know how many these creatures are.

When one sleeps, his doppelganger goes out of him and goes to the space. During that time the doppelganger is connected to the body only through a thread. If you wake somebody and startle him, his doppelganger does not manage to go back to his body, as result of which it entangles with other doppelgangers in the space. If one does not know how to disentangle

227

his doppelganger, he goes crazy.

Contemporary people are ailing, because they do not know how to eat, when to go to bed and when to get up. Many people get up at 4 a.m. That hour belongs to the Earth, which is why it is not convenient. If you get up at 2 a.m., this is the hour of the Moon. Again it is not convenient. Good hours are midnight, 1 a.m., 3 a.m., 5 a.m. and 6 a.m. Some people sleep a lot till 9 or 10 a.m. – this is extremely unhealthy.

Sleeping after the sunrise is as if one is put under a waterfall, the waves of which beat from above. Such is also the effect of the solar energy on the nervous system of people.

It is dangerous for someone to sleep during the day.

Saints sleep a little – one or two hours are enough for them, but for ordinary people, five hours of sleep are enough.

For now 7 hours of sleep are needed for you. 5 hours also could be satisfactory for you, but on the condition that you have a deep sleep.

It is not needed for a rational person to sleep for seven hours. For one person, who lives a regular life, three hours of deep sleep are enough for restoration of the power. This concerns people, who understand the laws of Nature. One, who understands one work, may finish it within three hours, and one, who does not understand it, will finish it for 12 hours.

There are people, who sleep per 8-10 hours; they think that this is good for them. Less, but healthy sleep. If you turn several times during the night from one side to the other, you have not slept well. Healthy sleep means to wake up on the side, on which you have fallen asleep.

For the one, who knows when to sleep, how much to sleep and how to sleep, sleep is a blessing. If one cannot obey certain rules during sleeping, one sleeps without benefiting from it.

Normal sleep is when you lie on your right or on your left side without turning till the morning; when there is no snoring, moving, and when breathing is smooth and silent. It is best if you sleep on your right side; middling – on the left side, bad – on the back, and even worse – on the stomach.

It is correct one to sleep on his right side, but he also may sleep on his left side, when the energies on the surface of the Earth are positive, one shall lie on his left side, which is negative, in order normal exchange of the powers to take place. When the energies on the surface of the Earth are negative, one shall lie on his right side. Therefore one shall know if the energies on the surface of the Earth are positive or negative. In addition, the energy of the Earth is not the same everywhere. One shall know these powers and conform to them.

In order one to be in harmony with the cosmic flows, the head during a sleep, shall be turned to the north or to the east.

The yawn shows that certain powers and energies are at a standstill in someone. Yawn, as a natural process, is for restoration of a certain order of things. New energy is introduced in somebody at each yawning.

Never lie on your back, or if you do so, keep your mind awake. You may lie on your back, but your mind shall be concentrated, and do not all asleep, because the vital powers, which flow along the spinal column, cannot function properly and the nerves are being pressed

When you go to bed in the evening, dress a clean shirt. Do not remain with the one, which have gathered dirt during the whole day.

In the evening, when one goes to bed, he has to fence well – his house, his bed, his body, as well as all parts of his organism. This was done by people since old times, by prayers and songs. Today you go to bed and say the formula: "There is no Love like God's one. Only God's Love is Love."

You can lie down at mountain areas, but without falling asleep. You shall choose, if possible, the south and east slopes, which are healthy and have accumulated energy from the blue color.

When a disciple makes a mistake, it is well, for several nights, to sleep on pine boards, without a pillow, to take in the qualities of the pine. The pine introduces an impulse for growth upwards and at the same time softens the character.

People, who exercise in occult science, renovate themselves and develop spiritually their bodies, by leaving their physical bodies on the Earth in the evenings and going out of the zone of the Earth for a mountain walk by the spiritual one. They renovate there and after that go back to their bodies. This is one method for a rest. People go to a resort, for a walk, but if they knew that method for renovation, they could use it. That method may be used also during the day: you will go under a tree, lean on it, go out of your body and after a walk, you will go back, but already renovated with fresh powers and health.

Clothing

Each article of clothing is a conductor of certain energy. Man shall know what type of energy he needs and through what kind of clothing he may provide it to himself, which clothes are conductors of the light and which are not.

The clothes of the reasonable person should be made of plant material. Wool clothes, made of the wool of sheep, are to be recommended to some extent, too.

Best clothes for education are linen and cotton ones. Wool clothes are good for poor people. Clothes shall be sewn without lining. If you are healthy and wear such a wool garment, magnetic coating is formed instead of lining between the body and the garment, which does not let external cold through. Even the thinnest garment, penetrated by magnetism, keeps warm.

Linen clothes are the best conductors of the electrical and magnetic energies. Wool clothes, under the present conditions, are the most hygienic, then the cotton ones come, but the best ones are the hemp and linen clothes.

You'd better not wear leather caps and rubber boots.

When you deal with spiritual matters, you shall be dressed in linen clothes.

Hemp clothing is also good.

Clothing should be wide in order permanent airing to take place and the electric and magnetic flows to pass freely. Clothing should be light.

Then, you shall turn attention to your hats and your hair. If you buy a hat, you shall take care it to be knobby, without many folds. When a person folds his hat, his character folds, too.

Perceiving of the higher energies cannot happen through an animal skin. The brain cannot perceive enough food and energy from above and the sense of refinement through the leather caps.

Never wear new clothes over old ones.

Wear clothes with one color, light, not many-colored. They could be stripes or spotted at the most. Wear nice and modest clothes.

Having in mind the present development of the mankind, it is best people to dress in clothes that have soft and pleasant colors to soften their feelings. Many people wear laces or clothes in bright inappropriate for them colors that are harmful to their nervous system.

The new study does not allow one and the same article of clothing to be worn two days on the run. Your clothes should not have the same colors. Each suit shall have a different color.

Sleeves are to be wide, and dresses - long.

Knowing that the old clothes were soaked with infectious microbes, with bad thoughts and feelings, with negative states, throw them or burn them, but never give them to the poor.

Rule: Do not give your clothes as a gift to somebody else. If you want to give, you are to buy something new.

If you have been ill for a long time in a dress, no matter how nice and expensive it is, throw it.

When someone is ill, he shall dress in white. One, who is healthy, shall change the colors. The flowers evoke movement, life, therefore you should change them.

There shall be space of half a millimeter between the shoe and foot, and the heel shall not be higher than 3-4 cm.

Shirts of healthy people should be sewn or knit by golden needles. Iron needles introduce something disharmonious in the character.

Hair

Each hair is a conductor of the light. You do not even suspect what relation hairs have to the external powers of Nature. That is why hairs should be kept always in a good state, combed, in order these powers to flow properly through you. If you do not feel well, if you are depressed and your things do not go well, do not go from house to house to complain, but run fingers through your hair. Do this useful exercise at least three times a day.

Short hair has electricity and magnetism, and the long one - magnetism. One may have short or long hair. One, who wants to develop his mind, under certain conditions, he may have short hair. Long hair shows the health state of the organism.

Long hair holds more electricity and magnetism. Having cut his hair, one is deprived of that energy. I do not approve hair cutting. It is well if hair reaches the length of at least the lower part of the ear.

If a person has gathered much magnetism in him, it is better to cut his hair. It is even healthy for him. Short hair introduces more electricity in the organism.

Take care, if possible, your hair to be tidied. While falling from the head every hair forms a certain angle. These angles of the hairs play a very important role in the refraction of the light. You may consider these things rather petty, but know that life is related only to small things.

One tip: during combing, do not throw away hairs that fall, but collect them in a bag. When you gather a lot, take them to Vitosha and burn them there on a clean stone. Let the ash from the hairs spread throughout the air in order ideas, which have passed through your head, to be fertilized.

Instead of an umbrella, Nature has put hair. When the light falls on the head, hairs distract it and it becomes harmless. If you carry an umbrella to protect yourself against the sun, you are deprived of the solar energy.

It is well if you often wet your hair with pure mountain water, but not to wash it, especially with soap, because it contains fat. Bring a comb with straight teeth and comb your hair often. If you often direct your thought toward the hairs, especially to the roots, your hairs strengthen and grow for one year. Hair loss is due to inner restlessness and lack of moisture in the organism.

When you wash your head, you shall wash it with soap only once a month, but with a nice clean soap. Otherwise, you can often wash your head, but without soap – only with water or with pure medicinal clay. You shall bake the medicinal clay well; add a little vinegar and plenty of water. You shall put from this mixture several times on your head and then wash it with clean water. In this way hair becomes soft and retains its magnetism. Fat is needed for the hair. If you wash it a lot, it becomes dry, electric. If the head is well washed, the skin breathes well, but you will deprive of the warmth and activity of the brain. With the loss of magnetism, human thinking capacity is reduced. Do not wear a hat, through which there is no airing of the head. When you get up in the morning, wet a little your head with warm water, according to the body temperature. Then comb the hair. If you yourself may make a soap, which will be of the best oil, then you may wash your hair more often. Contemporary soaps are not pure. They are made of dead animals. Medicinal clay is preferable to soap. You should not wash your head neither with very cold water, nor with hot water. You will get rid of the dandruff from your hair, if you live normally.

I would recommend you to always carry one comb in your pocket and your hair to always be at the back. This will help you a lot with regards to the health.

When the head is covered with hairs, then magnetism functions very well, and when the head goes bald, people get nervous.

People have tried lots of methods for restoring their hair. You, by concentrating your mind, say: "God, let my hair grow and thicken a little" and you will have a result sooner than by the other methods. Most often hair loss is due to anxiety.

Hair loss is due to anxieties, fears, and faults.

Sometimes hair turns gray also as a result of too much knowledge, but, most often, of big concerns. Sometimes hair turns grey from nonsense, sometimes of great intelligence. It may turn grey in 24 hours, but it may turn black also in 24 hours.

Why do the hairs on your head grow? When the warmth in man is bigger, the hairs on his head grow. When the warmth begins to decrease, hairs fall.

Once a person loses his magnetism, hair falls. If the warmth is more than it is needed, your hair will be curled, wrinkled. People, whose hair is too wrinkled, are very stubborn.

If you lived a quiet life, your hairs could grow such as they have to be. If you touch the hair of a holy person, this will give you peace. The saint has gathered energy from the Sun.

If you do not feel well, fondle your hair and you will immediately feel power and comfort. If you think good, you will have nice hair. Think good to change the hairs on your head.

Spiritual Life

To avoid diseases, one must eat the fruits of the Spirit: Love, peace, joy, patience, gentleness, temperance, and mercy. If he does not eat them, he comes upon the negative powers of Nature. He experiences hatred, suspicion, suffering, and falls ill.

When one raises mentally and spiritually, he becomes physically healthy. Knowing this, work on you and become internally clean - in mind, heart, and deeds.

Thank for all blessings that are being give to you. Dissatisfaction is spiritual impurity, which blocks the pores of the human body. Clean of it in the way water cleans your pores, and opens 7 million pores, through which you breathe.

You cannot be healthy, have strong arms and legs, healthy eyes, nervous system, if you are not good.

One should be good to maintain the normal state of the heart. If he does not love, neither his heart will be healthy, nor will his blood circulation be normal. If he is not smart, i.e. if his mind is weak, the headache comes. In some areas of the brain, excess energy that is useless accumulates. By harnessing this energy to work, his headache will stop. Almost all diseases come from not loving.

There is no hygiene without Love.

The strength of man is not in his muscles, but in that delicate and tender feeling, which may develop all other powers. And God made the world so that Nature submits to a seemingly weak power - Love.

Love is able to regulate warmth and light in our inner life, to regulate the powers, acting in the human organism.

If you walk along the path of Love, Wisdom and Truth, you will be a master of death, a master of poverty, diseases, of everyone.

Many people complain of cold limbs. They are looking for a way to help themselves. Many methods may be applied - washing of the feet in hot water, quick movements, but these are external methods. To heal, one must find the reason for his painful or abnormal state of the body. Cold limbs are due to impure blood in the organism. Impure blood produces electricity in the organism, and the clean one - magnetism. Electricity produces cold, and magnetism - warmth. Therefore, in order your limbs not to get cold, you have to introduce into your organism more warmth. This happens when one unlocks the Divine in you. In such a case, he will not be afraid neither of cold, nor of poverty, nor of diseases.

When you get up in the morning, say: "God, bless all those, who are in me and outside me, to work for Your glory and greatness. Give us light to understand You will and do it."

Cells that live in humans are rational, intelligent beings. They have a lot of knowledge, but their master shall be smart to know how to rule them. In order to enter the human organism, they have deliberately deprived themselves of individuality. Their aim is to sacrifice for their master and thus raise him. Man enjoys life while these intelligent creatures are able to work with him for his good. If they give up on him, his life becomes a desert.

At the occult school it is not allowed people to fix each other. Do you think that you shall close that sewage, through which all dirt flow out? No, thus you will create the greatest misfortune for people. The man, who is angry, is a channel, so let all impurities flow out; do not stop him. At the moment when he is angry and says all sorts of words, he helps people in this way, because many impurities go out through him. Today he is on duty. Tomorrow you may be on duty.

If you want to be healthy, learn not to notice the negative and wicked deeds of people. Close your eyes for everything you consider incorrect. Even if you see the bad deeds, do not criticize them.

The prayer increases the vibrations of the human aura, and becomes invulnerable to the lower ambient influences through this.

While praying one receives energy from the Divine world. The law of the prayer is the same as the law of eating. When one deprives of food, he feels a certain lack. When the soul is deprived of the prayer, it also feels that something is missing.

There is nothing that man has asked God for and that is not fulfilled. And it happens just when one needs it.

When you get up in the morning, thank God that your head is in place, that the heart and your body are in place and start working with them.

Alpha and Omega of things are to thank.

Stand before God like a child and say: God, bless me. Thank You for everything that You have given me. Help me to increase the freedom of my soul, the power of my spirit, the light of my mind and the goodness of my heart."

In order not to catch a cold, one must fence himself. This is achieved in two ways: by concentrating of the mind and through a prayer. Some people think that prayer is an easily applicable method. It depends on what will be the prayer. If you pray mechanically, no result will be achieved. Therefore, a concentrated thought and a conscious prayer are conditions for human's fencing for avoiding bad external conditions. If one is fenced, he does not catch a cold and nothing may attack him from outside.

Here is how to read "Our Father". First, you will fill your lungs with air. You will take in the air from God and say: "God, thank You for the air." And you will begin: "Our Father, who is in Heaven." Then you will inhale again. Before each subsequent sentence you will inhale. Thus, you will see after how many breaths you will read the entire prayer "Our Father". In the morning you will read with inhalations, at noon - with inhalations, and in the evening, before sunset - again. You will say you have no time to read "Our Father". You will not read it, but the doctors will cut your stomach, take away one of the kidneys, will cut the tonsils, will cut the caecum, or take out a tumor.

The most favorable periods for praying are the hours from 10 p.m. to midnight and from 3 a.m. to 4 a.m.

One, who may connect to the Divine world, he will benefit of the healthy energies of Nature that raise and rejuvenate the human organism.

Lies, anger, hypocrisy, suspicion bears such an explosive substance that destroys the human organism. These are the powers that harden and age people.

Everyone may be completely healthy when there is unity between his thoughts, feelings, and deeds. If there are any contradictions, he shall say: "In the name of God, let all these contradictions and obstacles, put in my way to impede me, go to their places!"

One, who lies, introduces poison in his organism, which is stronger even than the real poison. That poison is transferred in the blood of future generations and they gradually degenerate.

When a person is happy with his life, always in good mood and grateful, he is open to the sky and closed for evil. One, who has faith and Love for God, will be in connection with the lofty world, from where he will receive everything, needed for his development.

Study Nature with Love to connect with its beautiful lines, with its colors, which help for the proper contraction and expansion of capillaries.

Strong lower feelings and influences are related to the liver. And if you do not control your lower feelings, you will upset your liver. And this will cause disorder to all other systems. Constant arguments, irritations, greediness, pride also upset the liver. A major internal worry, a big disappointment that blocks energies and a discouragement may crush someone. All these things may bring the worst diseases, decrease vibrations in lots of organs, spoil their normal functioning, change the chemical processes in them, and even change their anatomical structure. A healthy right thought is healthy. With a clean and right thought you may do miracles.

People and Their Environment

Air, water, food, light and warmth are the elements, through which the new science uses as methods for cardinal solving of life issues. One, who understands the properties and applications of these elements, may recover in 5 minutes.

You live in Nature, but you cannot profit from it. Why? You do not know its laws. If you want to be in harmony with it, to benefit from its wealth, start learning its language. In order to learn the language of Nature, you have to study the forms of the bodies, their content and meaning.

Every person benefits of the goods of Nature, depending on the degree of his development.

One shall live according to the laws of Nature. If he does not obey these laws voluntarily, Nature will compel him by force to obey them.

There are three sources, through which the Divine world influences us: through food that comes from the plant kingdom, through the air, which includes light, warmth, magnetism, and electricity, and through thoughts and feelings. Therefore, these are the three most important tributaries that constantly come from the Divine world. If you close any of these tributaries, you will find yourself in a great contradiction. So, one may perceive the Divine through food, through light, warmth, electricity, and magnetism, and finally through all the rest powers, acting in nature. One may perceive the Divine also through the most sublime and pure thought.

Enormous energy is locked in rocks, seas, Cosmos, and people have not yet used the full potential of their brains, nor have used these extraordinary sources of energy.

When talking about healthy, normal life, it means proper usage of the energies from the external world, from the rational Nature.

Once the digestive system is blocked, the respiratory is also blocked and breathing becomes rapid and irregular. That is why these two systems must be kept in good state. Eating, in general, means a process of perception: perception of the living powers of Nature. These powers are taken in through food, through the air, water, light, and warmth, and finally through the living thought. The rational man has ways, through which he may extract the living powers from these environments. One, who knows carbon, its properties and compounds, he may always extract life from it.

Do not think it is easy for one to cope with the powers, acting in Nature, as well as in every living being. If you touch a person, whose energies are opposite to yours, you will spoil your state. And then some time shall pass until you cope with these energies. For instance, it is not one and the same who will sew your clothes. Choose such a tailor, whose energies match yours. In other words, be friends with people, with whom you are in harmony. Use the services of those, with who you are in agreement and unity. In this respect, birds have solved this issue. To overcome difficulties in their lives, they have developed in themselves the art of sewing clothes by themselves, painting and arranging them by themselves. One must be careful when he chooses his tailor, cook, as well as the books he will read. It is not one and the same who the author is. It is better if you read the books of that author that suits your character. It is good to read books that author with whom you set up in a range. It is not important if these books will be scientific or fictional.

When the brain absorbs all energies, one becomes rough in his feelings. In order not to deprive of the opportunity to develop both the brain and the heart, one must properly distribute the energies of his organism. The good master distributes his wealth equally amongst all slaves. Therefore, a rational person distributes the energies equally between all organs. He sends to each cell as much energy as it is needed. Some people understand the purpose of the stomach in a wrong way and say that it must be destroyed. No! The stomach has its great purpose. Without a stomach, physical life is impossible. A stomach and a paunch are two different things. Paunch is the greedy human desires. If it comes to such desires, one must self-educate, but by no means he shall force his stomach.

As disciples, you have to study the powers of your organisms in order you to be able to influence them rationally. In addition, you should know the language of the cells, of which your organs are composed, and chat with them. The more intelligent and highly developed one is, the more intelligent the cells of his body are. Know that one cannot think, feel, and act randomly. Each disharmony in thoughts, feelings, and actions reflects on the cells, and from there, on the state of the whole organism. One has to take into account the good of his organism. If he does not think good of his body, his body also does not think good of him. One should not overload his organism, nor leave it idle. He shall work, rest, and eat moderately. If you have a close look at the work of your cells, you will see that between them there are chemists, scientists, professors that do their experiments, perform numerous complex reactions, which may not be done by a human being in any of his laboratories. After all this one thinks that he knows his organism or the organism of those below him.

If you want to forget some things, you shall introduce into yourself the black color and you shall dress in black. If you want to remember some things, you shall dress in white.

All, who deal with mental work, have excess energy, which, if not transform by physical labor, will create great evils. However, those, who are engaged in physical labor, often suffer with overwork, which creates other evils. We do not approve overworking, nor idleness.

When you are very close to each other, entanglement of your auras occurs and instead of helping, you impede each other.

When you sit down, there shall be at least one meter between you in order not to entangle your auras. It is enough your spiritual body to come out of your at 2-3 mm for you to tolerate. It is sensitive and feels the opposite vibrations.

Besides the bad smell that comes out of the human body when it sweats, there is another influence that flows out from man, one impure matter that you cannot see and that is why you say: "I cannot understand why, but I cannot stand that man." The influence is bad. Sometimes something unpleasant comes out from the eyes.

God has determined the measure, at which we may approach each other. The hand is the measure. You give your hand forward for a handshake, as well as the other person – this is the natural position. There shall be no pulling or pressing of hands.

There shall be only slight shaking and a small holding of hands, thumbs always on top. The thumb shall not be bent down, and the hand shall be stretched, not bent. You shall cover the whole wrist, and not just a few fingers. Some people even handshake only with one or two fingers. It is very ugly. You will either shake hands or not. You may raise hand in greeting, in which case the hand is bent at the elbow, and the palm with folded fingers is completely directed toward your friend.

You may meet somebody with thick, magnetic, and electrical vibrations, filled with mud. You cannot easily get rid of that mud and a headache appears.

There are people, who, only if you look at them, bring bad luck to you. These are spiritual attacks. So, you shall study the powers, acting within you and outside of you. Now you study only the results. You do not like somebody, but this is a result.

Stay at least at one meter from each other. Do not approach too much each other. I have said that to you lots of times. Obey that rule.

Women get older of too much love. Their teeth fall of too much love. Their eyes weaken of too much love, of course, of the misunderstood love.

Women shall not wait and seek for the love of the others. She herself is a source, from which love shall spring. She shall loves. There is no need for her to wait to be loved.

High peaks are dynamic centers. They represent a reservoir of powers that will be used in the future. Mountain peaks are associated with the center of the Sun. At the same time, they are pumps that draw out impurities. For example, if you do not feel well and go up on a mountain peak, your discomfort will disappear and you will return refreshed and renewed. People do not feel well down in the valley. They feel depressed and tense there. Once you climb the mountain, the discomfort disappears.

It is good to go on excursions whenever it is possible from 14 January to 14 June, because within that period Nature is full of the vital prana at most.

The power of people is not only in physical food. To be strong, one must know how to use the air that he breathes, to send it to all cells of the lungs, in order breathing to be proper. In order to be strong, one shall know how to regulate the flows of his sympathetic nervous system, particularly the solar plexus and cerebellum. To be strong, one shall know how to regulate the energies of his stomach. Finally, knowing how to manage the lungs, the sympathetic nervous system and the stomach, a person will begin to study the brain, i.e. the real person.

The woman shall be stronger in the astral world, and the man shall be stronger in the mental world. If a woman has entered into the love of a man, she shall feel a pleasant coolness, released from him toward her, after she has been heated in her warmth up to 45 degrees. Under the warmth of a woman everything grows and develops. And for the understanding and application of love coolness is required, thanks to which fruits do not spoil.

Many ideas fail, because love of women has no vibrations with such warmth as it should be, and love of men has no such coolness as it is necessary. Speaking of men and women, I mean the human himself.

If a person falls ill of grief over somebody beloved, and because the center of love is behind, temperature raises due to love. Why does one fall ill? One thinks of his/her beloved and wants to have her/him constantly beside him/her.

Nature never allows what it has given you to be obsessed. It gives you something to use it, but not obsess it. If you do so, it always counteract. If you want to conquer what it has created, you will create a painful condition for yourself.

You have the right to love, but you do not have the right to obsess. You have the right to eat, but you do not have the right to overeat. You have the right to cry, but not crying out loud or screaming. Cry quietly. Someone is sitting somewhere and his tears are falling and after crying for a while, he feels better. Someone else roars and is heard for miles - this is bad crying. God loves the quiet, humble, broken heart. I am glad when someone cries, but it is not good crying for more than 10 minutes. Saturday is the only day when crying is not allowed. Sunday is a free day - then you may cry. There shall be no crying on the day of God. You shall be happy and joyful from morning to night. On Saturday you will work for God. You will not cry then, but thank. Someone says: "How may I be happy in that poverty?". You have to enjoy poverty, too.

We have normal and healthy lives, when we spend the energies of our organisms properly and when the external energies, the energies of the Rational Nature, are taken in properly. There is something in man that is prone to sin, due to which Nature has implemented the ability of modifying in the matter. Scientists say that the human body reconstructs at intervals of seven years. Each seven years the bone, muscle, nerve and brain tissues renovate. Others say that one may renovate within three months - it depends on his thoughts and feelings. It is enough one to commit only one crime to stain the matter of his body. To rebuild his body, one shall have clean as a spring life, which shall constantly spring and clean itself.

Once the weight center of the human brain goes to the back of the head, life also becomes hard, and to make it easier, one may pass the flows from the back part of the brain to the front part and thus change his states. Sometimes the electrical and magnetic flows in the organism go perpendicularly to the spine, due to which a severe shock to the brain takes place. This may be noticed with people who, while walking, hit their heels and distort their shoe heels.

Do not allow any hump on your body. It interrupts the flow of the energies from the sympathetic nervous system to the brain.

Somebody may say that he does not need knowledge of astronomy or biology, or physics, chemistry, mathematics, psychology, etc. You do need all sciences. You shall study all sciences, as well as electricity and magnetism, because they are powers, operating in the organism.

If every morning from the middle of May, June till the middle of July, before sunrise, you worked only for half an hour in your garden, you would be healthy. Then there is an earth energy that comes from the southern hemisphere and goes to the northern one, makes a whole circle, then goes back to the southern hemisphere. Growth, blossoming, creating of forms, fruits depend on that energy. All people suffer with deficiency of that energy, because they do not want to communicate with the earth, and an exchange between man and the earth is needed. Dirt, mud, weeds from your organism shall go down into the earth in order fresh powers to go up in you.

Modern people need a new understanding of things, with which to reconstruct the brain, lungs, stomach, and the muscle system. Until he rebuilds his organs, one may not properly perceive the light that comes from the Sun.

The more solar energy you take in yourself, the greater softness and magnetism will be developed in you, and then, everybody will love you.

If you want your heart to be healthy, you shall keep your brain, from where electric flows of Nature pass, and the solar plexus, from where the magnetic flows pass, in good state.

The early rays are the most favorable to people. There is a large transformer in the Sun that sends energy throughout the Earth. There is also a specific transformer for every person on Earth in the Sun. Everyone accepts the specially sent to him light and energy. Everyone has a transformer that accepts that special light, sent for him.

The larger the windows at home and the more often they are open, the more healthy people are.

The windows of your home shall be large for light to come in freely.

Expose yourself to the sun, to connect with God.

If you want to be healthy, to physically and spiritually develop normally, take care of the state of the capillaries. They shall contract and expand properly. For that purpose, never drink cold ice water. If you drink cold water, the capillaries of the throat and stomach contract too much and cause numerous painful states. Never breathe through the mouth, because the capillaries of the lungs contract. Take the air through the nose for it to clean and warm.

It is dangerous for people when the capillaries expand more than it is needed, without being able to contract. It is also dangerous when they contract more than it is needed, without being able to expand.

Always drink warm water or if it is cold, drink slowly, with alert consciousness. Eat foods that you love. Sleep in a room that you love. When you get up in the morning always do this on the right side of the bed. Sleep on the right side, and your head shall be to the north or east.

Never pour water, with which you have washed your face, at unclean places. It is good for the unclean places, but it is not good for you. This water shall be thrown at the flowers, the trees, but never at places, where people pass or at unclean places. Follow that rule, do not ask why, and you will improve.

The water you drink shall not be chalky. Hard water leaves lots of sediments.

The program of all religious systems as a method of work it is recommended people to grow plants. One treats through them. By taking care of them, one becomes familiar with their magical power. Everyone shall have in his garden a few beds of garlic, onion, parsley, which to grow with care and love.

You shall not avoid working with the earth. Every plant, every fruit, with which one deals, introduces its qualities in him. It is good for you to grow an india-rubber plant. It is a fruitless plant, but gives something from itself. One, who wants to get rich, shall grow an india-rubber plant, which also introduces calmness and good mood. It is for educated people. If you want to become active, vigorous, grow cherries, mainly red. If you want to strengthen your faith, grow plums. Through plants you may treat yourself. They contain a magical power. Nowadays, garlic is especially recommended as a remedy.

In the morning, the solar energy is mother's love, and in the afternoon, energy degenerates, becomes bad, and in the evening and at night, it is even worse.

When you do not feel well, do not touch my eyebrows. Touching them is a sacred act - they are the boundary between the astral and the Divine world.

You shall walk barefoot in summer, especially at the beginning of May, so that your feet to be in connection with the earth and electricity and earth magnetism to go into you. Those of you, who are not used to barefoot walking, shall walk barefoot just for 1-2 hours after the sunrise. This is nice. I would recommend to both men and women to go out barefoot at sunrise, but outside the city, within a nice place.

It is good from time to time one to be barefoot, because, through the legs as antennas, he comes in contact with the earth. Between the energies of the earth and his energies a proper exchange takes place. However, there are hours during the day and hours during the year when this exchange is not needed. There are days and hours, when you can walk barefoot, but there are days and hours, when it is by no means allowed people to be barefoot.

Your future depends on the way you sit. You are sitting and you are constantly changing your position. You put your left leg on the right one, and vice versa. You are rotating constantly and bending your spine.

You consider that of no importance, but I tell you, it is very important how one sits, how he moves, how he works, how he starts off. By the way, in which one sits, his character may be identified.

Gold maintains the health of the organism. Gold is a good conductor of warmth and electricity. Therefore, organic gold in the human blood is a conductor of energies in Nature.

Human organism needs a variety of items, and not just gold. Gold bears the vital energies of Nature, and silver cleans people of impurities in the organism. Iron strengthens the organism. However, if one introduces more iron in the organism than needed, he becomes rough. Each element has its purpose for the human organism, but only if it is used in a certain amount.

Precious stones are bearers of ascending creative energies and serve as natural transformers. Therefore, it is recommended precious stones to be worn as a shield against harmful influences and as transformers of lower desires.

Approach everything that God has created – flowers, fruit trees. To be healthy, plant some flowers in pots or in your garden and take care of them. Plant fruit trees and vegetables in your garden to study them and benefit of their powers. Get into contact also with the sunrays.

One, who wants to be healthy, not to suffer, let him grow flowers. They heal, revive, and rejuvenate people.

Love plants and forests to connect with the powers, acting in them. They are a warehouse of powers, from where one may draw what he needs for his body.

Why do the branches of some trees bend? If in somebody's garden there are such trees, the owner has wicked thoughts and feelings. These wicked thoughts and feelings form improper mind waves, which are absorbed by the ether doppelganger of the plants and branches bend. This also concerns animals. The ferocity of beasts in the mountains and in woods increases by bad and ferocious thoughts and feelings of the people, which they adopt in their astral body. People have one responsibility for that.

Do not plant trees exactly next to your house. Plants inadvertently do harm to you. There is a thirst for water in plants. If you lie down under a walnut or fall asleep under another tree, you will see what they can do. They pull out the juices of life.

Even if you are ill, if you love flowers, you will recover soon. Flowers regulate the nervous system. It is good for someone nervous to water red flowers and smell them.

Eating without the involvement of the mind is not healthy. The way thoughts, feeling, and deeds are inseparable, thinking, breathing and eating shall be connected in the same way.

Take light, air, water and food consciously and with love to benefit from them, to have good results. If you take them just as mechanical goods, you will have poor results. While breathing, think that in the air besides oxygen and nitrogen, there is something else that brings life. While drinking water, think that besides hydrogen and oxygen, there is something else that brings life in it. Generally, any compound, any fruit has life in itself.

Good thoughts maintain the good states of the brain health, good feelings – the proper blood circulation and breathing, and good deeds – the health of the stomach system.

Beware of strong winds and flows. There are strong winds and warm flows that are dangerous to humans, because they take out the moisture from their bodies. Quiet winds are nice for air baths.

To improve people's lives and their health, it is recommended for all external and internal purity. Purity is able to keep human health, to keep the energy and continue his life.

It is required everybody to have physical, heart, and mental purity. On the streets, at home or in the mountains, everywhere, one must keep absolute purity. One, who consciously maintains the purity of the physical life, he will be clean in the heart and mental lives. It is not possible one to speak of a high ideal, of faith in God, if he does not keep the simplest purity of the physical world. One shall be clean in every respect!

Do not allow anyone to enter your home with muddy or dusty shoes. You will make them take off their shoes and then enter.

As long as one has come to Earth, he must start with the physical cleanness. Clothes, shoes, the body must be perfectly clean. One shall wash his face, hands, and teeth ten times a day. Teeth should not be always washed with a brush. It is enough to wash them with warm water and soap or with a little alcohol. Many diseases are due to microbes that develop in the teeth. If one is not prepared to maintain physical cleanness of the body, how he will maintain his spiritual purity?

Health without purity is unachievable, every cell in you shall be clean externally and internally. The overall purity of the cells is also purity of the body. In the future, your bodies will change.

One, who deals with people's dirt, corrupts. If you have physical purity, you will also have spiritual one. Physical and spiritual purities are necessary for creating a favorable atmosphere for the human mind. By impurity of thoughts, an unpleasant atmosphere is created, from which people demagnetize.

Doubt is some sort of impurity, which enters the astral body and one feels envy, fear, and hatred. One, who wants to have a new body, shall kept clean his physical, astral (star), and mental body and keep a link between them.

Once the impure matter (e.g. from a furuncle) comes out of somebody, the discomfort disappears, and it shall be by all means be thrown out. All low thoughts and desires in man shall be thrown out and only healthy thoughts and feelings shall remain in him.

The only salvation of man from microbes is pure blood. When blood is absolutely clean, man resists all microbes. Even if they go in his blood, there are no conditions for them to multiply. When we say that a man must be absolutely clean, with high moral, we mean those favorable conditions, which protect him from microbes. Purity protects people from those invisible, secret enemies, who introduce the most powerful poisons in the organism.

The new morality requires absolute purity from all: purity of the body – of all external and internal organs; purity in thoughts, feelings, and deeds. Purity in veins and arteries, purity in blood. You all shall have absolutely clean blood.

Pure life provides pure blood. The organism of modern people is infected by meat, wine and lots of other foods. Our spiritual body is infected by greed, anger, hatred. You love someone, but when he says something bad to you, you begin to hate him. Do you know what a dangerous poison hatred is for your organism? In that case you do harm to yourself. Pride is also a poison.

When one deals exclusively with people's mistakes he comes to the state to attract toward himself astral bacteria that upset his organism. To deal with the mistakes of people, this means to connect with them and bear the bad effects of these mistakes. Every evil thought, every bad feeling attracts attracts lower beings accordingly. So you shall also observe hygiene of the mind, heart, and soul. Christ said: "Keep your eyes clear to be clean your whole body." Purity, holiness, love - this is the hygiene of the soul. The application of love in life is that state of health of the human organism, at which one may fulfill his purpose.

You shall not judge anybody on Saturday. On Saturday you shall become deeply absorbed in yourself, you shall think, pray, sing, be a master of your position.

You will put on your best clothes.

People influence each other. If you live amongst ill people, you will experience their state. If you live amongst healthy people, you will be healthy. Under that law, one shall wish in his soul to have a healthy body, noble feelings, and bright thoughts. One shall wish his relatives and friends the same.

Do not go to your friend if you are ill, angry, or bitter. Go into the forest, call at trees, stones, and complain to them. When your mind is calm and your heart free, then visit your friend.

Do not go to people's homes when you feel wretched to share your grief in order to feel better! Do not bring your waste to the others. Do not load them with your weights.

Do not rely on the services of nervous oppressive people no matter if it is for sewing, for making shoes, a house, etc. Never allow a nervous and dry person to cook for you. The person, who cooks for you shall be stout, healthy and cheerful. People, who are very dry, do not have that sublime spiritual understanding, are not from the Divine world, for the simple reason that they contain lots of acid, from which large activity occurs. And stout people are like foundations.

Do not allow someone, who is ill or bad to touch you. If a healthy person puts his hand on you, he will give you something.

There are people, who should not be close to each other. It is due to the fact that one of them is heated to thousands of degrees and is made of iron, and the other next to him is made of wood. Do not sit too close to each other to avoid doing harm to each other.

Do not sit to someone, who does not love you, or to someone, whom you do not love, either.

The state of feelings and thoughts raises by reading books which describe the life and works of the saints, of great people. When discouragement comes, do not be afraid. You have come temporarily in that sphere, where creatures attack you with their thoughts and feelings in order to rob you. They are thieves and robbers, who have in mind your discouragement. Keep your mind alert to be able to cope easily with them.

The airplane and the car are means for moving people from one place to another. In the same way the cat may be a means for someone to manifest himself. One creature may come in and go out of the cat in the way you come in and go out of a car. Animals are a vehicle for human underdeveloped souls.

Knowledge is the material, thanks to which consciousness is purified, and consciousness feeds and maintains the mental body. If you cannot learn, acquire knowledge, the mental body will go away.

You must keep your body from being burnt, from massages with gas, iodine, and other medicines. The skin shall be kept in a soft state, because the pores are the lungs, through which the soul breathes in the physical world.

When some people feel weak and anemic, use artificial cosmetics for making themselves beautiful. Women use lipsticks and powders, but, as a result of this, their skin soon wrinkles and instead of becoming beautiful, they do themselves harm. There is internal cosmetics - clean thoughts and feelings, and noble deeds.

The life of modern people is full of worries and embarrassments. If they have a headache, they embarrass. If they have a stomachache, rheumatism, they embarrass. One shall not worry and embarrass, but give. Give selflessly to get rid of the painful states.

Every bad word or thought, addressed to you, is a psychological bomb that explodes in you and causes some destruction. In order physical or mental destructions not to happen, you shall have in your mind and heart good thoughts and feelings for yourself, as well as for the others.

Anger, rage, lust are negative qualities, in which there is no intelligence, and love and humility are the original virtues, with which man was created and they are the intelligent powers that raise. In anger and rage you demagnetize and fall low.

Ill feelings are wastefulness. Thousands of cells die in each ill feeling or rage. Sometimes 4-5 million of blood cells become victims to anger. Neurasthenia is a constant irritation; the energy that originates is not used properly and is not put in place. That energy may be sent in the upper centers of the brain, in front or on top of the head.

Doubt, suspicion, jealousy, and envy are mental microbes. Put them away from you if you want to be healthy.

The Bible presents rules, methods, and ways of rational living in every respect. There is a book, in which all ideas and rules on how one must live are set out.

One should be neither too fat, nor too thin. There are normal measures that you need to meet. The neck shall be twice wider than the size of the hand. By taking into consideration the dimensions of the body in relation to the hand, you may guess which way you are on. One has to work on his physical body and gradually go to his spiritual body. Furthermore, by touching the hand, depending on its normal warmth, you may guess what the state of health of the organism is. If your hand is cold or hot more than it is needed, this shows that the state of the organism is not normal. If you feel any abnormal state of your organism, take measures to improve it: spend 1-2 days in fasting, drink more hot water, breathe fresh air and expose yourself to light.

Never leave your larynx to go through sudden conditions – from cold to hot and vice versa. Sour and spicy foods spoil your voice. Eat sweet foods for good voice.

For a disciple, physical, mental, and spiritual work must be equally sacred.

For a saint 1 hour is determined for physical work, 3 hours - for the heart and 7 hours – mental work. And some of you do not work. And now, due to idleness, deformation in the organisms starts. You begin to feel pain in the head, the stomach, the legs, the arms. It is good to have a garden, where to work for at least one hour to get rid of the useless energy. You will dig with a hoe if you want to be healthy. There are negative energies, which have to enter in the earth.

Overeating in the physical, spiritual, or mental worlds, leads to surfeit. It is not allowed surfeit in work, either. Surfeit also leads to numerous painful diseases.

You need healthy food, no drinks or syrups, but only clean water, healthy clothes, homes with large windows, abundance of light, and at least two hours of physical work every day. The oils and pans shall be thrown away from your kitchen. It is a sin a woman to cook for 4-5 hours! What a culture is that? One hour is well enough for the preparation of the food, and the rest of the time shall be spent for spiritual work: reading, music, art and everything that can raise and ennoble the heart and soul.

Soap is not necessary for people. Once a month it is enough for one to wash with soap. The face has the ability to wash by itself. Electricity and magnetism flow out from each cell and pore of the body, which wash both the face and the whole body.

Modern people began to suffer with not-coming-out to a walk in the open air. We live like prisoners. Do you think that a building of 4-5 floors or 10 is healthy?

If someone lives for a long time in the mountain, he will gain something for sure or lose much. He will become wild and rougher. If he lives for a long time in the valley is not good, either. There shall be changes. There shall be coming up and down.

When you are on a walk in the mountain, go slowly, calmly, without haste. Stop at every one hundred meters for a short break of about 30 seconds per foot. The higher you climb, the slower you shall go. In this way you will adjust to the powers of Nature and you will use them wisely.

Throw away the black glasses from your eyes! One has to look right through his eyes, clearly, without obstructions. The soul is open and free to enjoy everything.

Behind each flower, there is a rational being stays, due to which it is not allowed they to be picked. It is allowed in an extreme case for remedy after the permission of the rational being.

Flowers, trees, vineyards, wheat fields have a beneficial impact on people, so I recommend you to visit them.

Trees are clean, flowers are clean, so when a criminal touches them, they wither, they die.

If you take care of fruit trees, they will introduce their qualities into you. People would be in trouble if they were no plums, cherries, pears, and all fruits. Plants are children of the angels, and if you deal with plants, you deal with angels. If you deal with the animals, you deal with cherubim and seraphim.

A farmer, who plows the field and when he reaps it, he shall use no bad words. There shall be only joy and songs. Wheat grains will be full of energy then. There is bread that heals.

Why do you tread on each caterpillar that appears on your way? One day it will become a butterfly, but you stop its evolution by squelching it. You stop the development process, but at the same time, you stop your own development process.

Human skin shall be soft, smooth and receptive. It is a regulator of life. If it becomes rough, one is jeopardized, easily gets ill, and dies earlier. The skin shall be neither dry, nor wet. Sorrows, pains, negative feelings like anger and envy roughen the skin and it may not take in the vital energy, prana so properly. In order the skin to be soft, clean, nice, it should not be used various ointments, but a special food that you will find and master.

One, who eats well, breathes properly, feels right, and thinks right, will always be healthy. One, who is not satisfied with eating, does not breathe, does not move, does not think right, and will always be ailing.

Health is determined by the hygiene that one keeps in the physical, heart and mental lives. Hygiene in the physical world requires people to know how to eat, drink, and breathe, and finally to know how to sleep.

To comply with the hygiene of the physical world, consider the three elements - home, food, and clothing; to comply with the hygiene of the spiritual world, consider the other three elements - thoughts, feelings, and deeds.

In the world there are people, clean and bright, that radiate from themselves a special inner power that feeds humans as physical food does. One might be well fed not only by physical food, but also by air and light. The air is taken through the pores, and in order pores to be opened, one should fast and sweat.

Divine world is not only fasting, torturing of the body, distortion of the mind and heart, but it is also an absolute harmony. You shall eat without overeating, sleep without oversleeping, dress up without excesses.

If you take the width of the neck and multiply it by two, you get the dimension of the waist. And if you get the width of the wrist and multiply it by the two, you get the width of the neck. Once these measures are breached, a person breaches the laws of Nature. Human health depends on the observance of these laws.

What will bring the stone house to man? Nothing, but misfortunes and sufferings. He must live at least 20 years in it to remake the rough material from which it is made.

It is easy to process the rough and low matter and turn it into finer. The body is also a house, but the better the matter, from which it is made, is organized, the healthier one is.

The healthiest homes are those that are made of trees, then the ones made of bricks come, and stone buildings are at the end. The healthiest homes are the ones made of glass.

Wooden houses are healthier than the stone ones. A house made of old trees transfer something valuable to people. If you are weak and painful, go out early in the morning and lean your back on an oak for 15-20 minutes to refresh.

A home must have at least three windows - to the east, to the south, and to the west, and these windows to be at least a meter and a half wide in order lots of light to be able to enter from outside. Homes shall not be square Corners are to be rounded for the atmosphere to be soft.

If someone has given you to eat something and he has put a bad thought in it, if you eat it, you will feel the thought and you will experience discomfort. In the past, people who knew these secrets of Nature, never wanted to eat bread, kneaded by a bad person, because they knew that there was something put in the bread, which was not good. This applies to everything given as a present. If your heart does not accept it, if it is not pleasant for you, do not accept it. I see that someone deliberately avoids walking along certain streets. He may use roundabout streets, but he shall pass through the streets, which are pleasant to him. May be the Earth flows do not correspond to his organism or the thoughts of the people, who live on those streets, are not in harmony with his ones – there always will be something. This is not a superstition. This is prevention. If you listen to your internal radio, it will tell you from where to pass, how to start off, etc. Nowadays, people do not listen to anything - they eat when they should not; sleep when they should not, and want to be healthy.

I tell Bulgarians not to be afraid, because they are the liver of mankind. If Bulgarians disappear, the liver will disappear, too. If the liver disappears, digestion cannot be performed properly. Each people performs a special work in the common Divine organism.

Ill people are not allowed in Heaven. They will ask you there: "Why are you ill? Didn't you have money, food, air, water? All this is given to you in abundance, but you have not used it properly. Come on now, go back to Earth to learn to use properly the blessings." Spiritual people must be absolutely healthy in body, heart, and mind.

Do you think that the light that is sent to you from the invisible world will not be taken into account? Do you think that the bread you have eaten or the energy you have used will not be taken into account? Every word of yours said in vain will be taken into account. Your life will be filmed in front of you in details to see how you wasted your time and how you spent your energy randomly.

It is all chronicled in the invisible world.

SONGS BY THE MASTER

For treatment and prevention of diseases of the liver, eyes, tendons, nervous system, and the bone system:

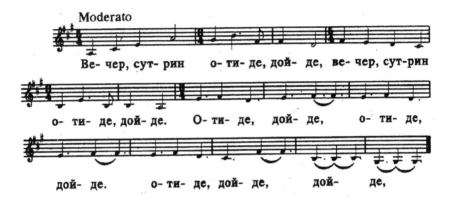

Transliteration:

Vecher, sutrin

Vecher, sutrin otide, doide,

vecher, sutrin otide, diode.

Otide, diode, otide, diode.

Otide, diode, diode.

Translation:

Evening, Morning

Evening, morning passed, came,

evening, morning passed, came.

Passed, came, passed, came.

Passed, came, came.

For treatment and prevention of diseases of the liver, eyes, tendons, nervous system, spleen, heart, mouth, muscles, and the blood vessels:

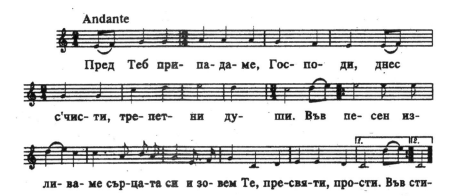

Пред Теб при- па- да- ме, Гос- по- ди, днес

с'чис- ти, тре- пет- ни ду- ши. Във пе- сен из-

ли- ва- ме сър- ца- та си и зо- вем Те, пре-свя-ти, про-сти. Във сти-

Transliteration:

Sardechen zov

Pred Teb pripadame, Gospodi, dnes

s chisti trepetni dushi.

Vav pesen izlivame sartsata si

i zovem Te, presvyati, prosti.

Zabravyai grehovete nashi,

obilno nas blagoslovi;

Tsaryu, Preblagii, na svetlite dushi

i v tsarstvoto Si ni priemi.

Tam da Te slavim prez vechnostta

edin Ti zasluzhavash hvala;

ogradi ni s milostite Si Tvoi,

ozari ni s Tvoita svetlina.

Translation:

Appeal of the Heart

Before You we bow down, God, today

with clean, eager souls.

In a song we unburden our hearts

and appeal You, Most Holy, forgive us.

Forget our sins,

and give us plenty of blessings;

You, Tsar, Most Kind, of the bright souls,

welcome us in Your Kingdom.

There we will glorify You eternally.

Only You deserve praise.

Fence us with Your grace,

light us up with Your light.

For treatment and prevention of diseases of the liver, eyes, tendons, nervous system, and the digestive system:

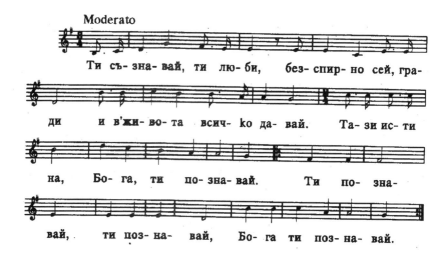

Transliteration:

Blagata pesen

Ti saznavai, ti lyubi,

bezspirno sei, gradi

i v zhivota vsichko davai.

Tazi istina, Boga, ti poznavai.

Ti poznavai, ti poznavai,

Boga ti poznavai.

Translation:

The Good Song

Be conscious, love,

sow unendingly, build,

and give everything in life.

Know that Truth, God.

Know, know

God. Know God.

For treatment and prevention of diseases of the kidneys, bone system, ears, and hair loss:

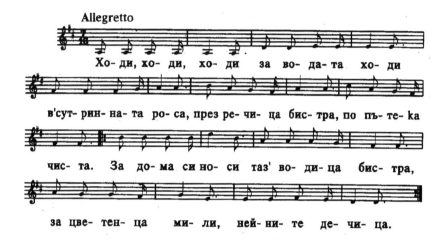

Allegretto

Хо- ди, хо- ди, хо- ди за во- да- та хо- ди

в'сут- рин- на- та ро- са, през ре- чи- ца бис- тра, по пъ- те- ка

чис- та. За до- ма си но- си таз' во- ди- ца бис- тра,

за цве- тен- ца ми- ли, ней- ни- те де- чи- ца.

Transliteration:

Hodi, hodi

Hodi, hodi za vodata, hodi v sutrinnata rosa,

prez rechitsa bistra, po pateka chista.

Za doma si nosi taz voditsa bistra,

za tsvetentsa mili, neinite dechitsa.

Translation:

Go, Go

Go, go for water, go at dew-fall,

through a clear river, along a clean path.

Bring home that clear water

for its small children – the flowers dear.

For treatment and prevention of diseases of the digestive system, kidneys, bone system, ears, and hair loss:

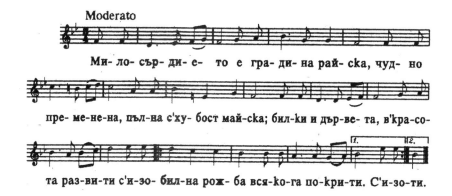

Transliteration:

Milosardieto

Milosardieto e gradina raiska,

chudno premenena, palna s hubost maiska;

bilki i darveta, v krasota razviti

s izobilna rozhba vsyakoga pokriti. (2)

Vsichko drago, milo i v lyubov zhivee

i tsafti, i varzhe, i raste, i zree.

Prolet, lyato, esen i prez tsyala zima,

ot kogato hora na zemyata ima. (2)

I stom patnik moren mine krai gradina,

vsyako zhivo klonche veselo mu kima;

Plodove uzreli bez korist predlaga

s neprestorna nega i usmivka blaga. (2)

Bedni i bogati, zdravi ili bolni,

i po vsyako vreme, tuka sa dovolni,

che smenyavat v radost grizhite – homota,

i s uteha vizhdat smisal vav zhivota. (2)

Zatui, koito diri istinska pobeda,

rai takav prekrasen neka si otgleda;

nyama da se svarshi shtastie za nego,

shte go blagoslavyat i zemya i nebo. (2)

Translation:

The Charity

Charity is a Paradise garden,

marvelously dressed up, full of May beauty;

herbs and trees in beauty developed,

and always well-laden. (2)

Everything lives in love, nicely and sweetly,

and blooms, and knits, and grows, and ripens.

In spring, in summer, in autumn and during the entire winter,

ever since there are people on the Earth. (2)

And when a tired traveler passes by the garden,

each living branch nods at him joyfully;

it offers mature fruits unselfishly

with unsophisticated bliss and a gentle smile. (2)

Rich and poor, healthy or ill beings

are always happy here

that they replace troubles in joy

and in consolation find sense in life. (2)

So, one, who looks for true victory,

paradise, so wonderful, let him grow by himself;

happiness will not end for him,

and he will be blessed by Earth and Heaven. (2)

For treatment and prevention of diseases of the digestive system, lungs, skin, nose, and allergies:

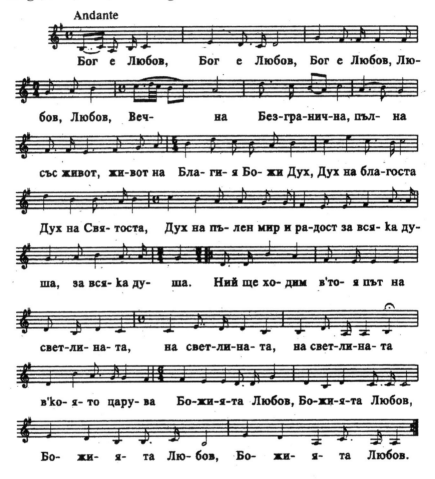

Transliteration:

Bog e lyubov

Bog e Lyubov, Bog e Lyubov, Bog e Lyubov,

Lyubov, Lyubov,

Vechna, Bezgranichna, palna sas zhivot,

zhivot na Blagia Bozhi Duh,

Duh na blagostta, Duh na svyatostta,

Duh na palen mir i radost

za vsyaka dusha, za vsyaka dusha.

Nii shte hodim v toya pat na svetlinata,

na svetlinata, na svetlinata,

v koyato tsaruva Bozhiyata Lyubov,

Bozhiyata Lyubov, Bozhiyata Lyubov, Bozhiyata Lyubov.

Translation:

God is Love

God is Love, God is Love, God is Love,

Love, Love,

Eternal, Boundless, full of life,

life of the Kind God's Spirit,

Spirit of Goodness, Spirit of Sacredness,

Spirit of complete peace and joy

for each soul, for each soul.

We will walk along that path of the light,

of the light, of the light,

where God's Love reigns,

God's Love, God's Love, God's Love.

For treatment and prevention of diseases of the gall-bladder, eyes, tendons, and headaches:

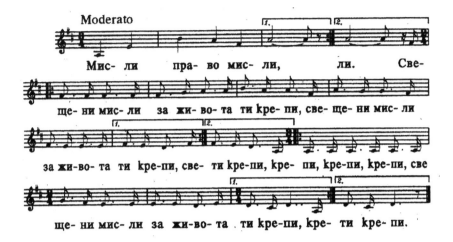

Transliteration:

Misli, pravo misli

Misli, pravo misli.

Sveshteni misli za zhivota ti krepi, (3)

krepi, (3)

sveshteni misli za zhivota ti krepi,

krepi, krepi.

Translation:

Think, Think Right

Think, think right.

Sacred thoughts of life you keep, (3)

keep, (3)

sacred thoughts of life you keep,

keep, keep.

For treatment and prevention of diseases of the heart, blood system, spleen, muscle system, mouth, liver, eyes, and the nervous system:

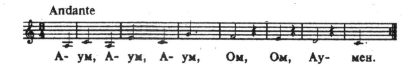

Transliteration & translation:

Aum

Aum, Aum, Aum, Om, Om, Aumen.

For treatment and prevention of diseases of the lungs, skin, nose, spleen, muscle system, mouth, and allergies:

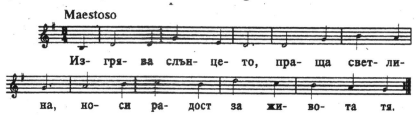

Transliteration:

Izgryava slantseto

Izgryava slantseto,

prashta svetlina,

nosi radost za zhivota tya.

Translation:

The Sun is Rising

The Sun is rising

and is sending light,

which brings joy to life.

For treatment and prevention of diseases of the heart, blood system, spleen, muscle system, and the mouth:

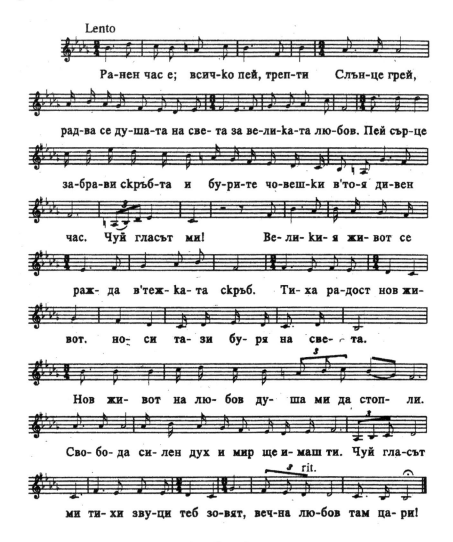

Transliteration:

Ranen chas

Ranen chas e;

vsichko pei, trepti.

Slantse grei,

radva se dushata na sveta za velikata lyubov.

Pei sartse, zabravi skrabta

i burite choveshki v toya diven chas.

Chui glasat mi!

Velikiya zhivot se razhda v tezhkata skrab.

Tiha radost, nov zhivot nosi tazi burya na sveta.

Nov zhivot na lyubov dusha mi da stopli.

Svoboda, silen duh i mir shte imash ti.

Chui glasat mi, tihi zvutsi teb zovyat,

vechna lyubov tam tsari!

Translation:

Early Morning

It is an early morning;

everything sings, vibrates.

The Sun is shining,

the soul enjoys the world for the Great Love.

Sing, heart, forget the sorrow

and the human storms at that glorious hour.

Listen to my voice!

Great life is born in the heavy sorrow.

Silent joy and new life are brought by that storm to the world.

Let my soul be warmed by a New life of Love.

You will have freedom and strong spirit.

Listen to my voice, silent sounds call you,

eternal love reigns there!

For treatment and prevention of diseases of the heart, blood system, gall-bladder, eyes, tendons, and headaches:

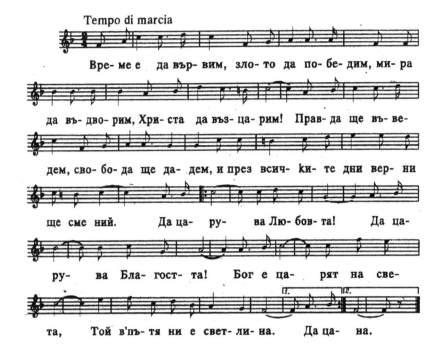

Transliteration:

Vreme e da varvim

Vreme e da varvim,

zloto da pobedim,

mira da vadvorim,

Hrista da vaztsarim!

Pravda shte vavedem,

svoboda shte dadem,

i prez vsichkite dni

verni shte sme nii.

Da tsaruva Lyubovta!

Da tsaruva Blagostta!

Bog e tsaryat na sveta,

Toi v patya ni e svetlina.

Barzo da poletim,

moshtno da vaztrabim,

radost da vazvestim,

vyara da sazhivim!

Shte ogrei pak sveta

v parva krasota,

svoboda, mir i red

shte vladeyat vred.

Da tsaruva Lyubovta!

Da tsaruva Blagostta!

Bog e tsaryat na sveta,

Toi v patya ni e svetlina.

Translation:

It is Time to Go

It is time to go,

to defeat evil,

to bring peace,

to enthrone Christ!

We will establish justice,

give freedom,

and during all days

we will be loyal.

Let Love reign!

Let Goodness reign!

God is Tsar of the world,

He is Light along our paths.

Let us fly forth quickly,

proclaim loudly,

herald joy,

and bring to life faith!

The world will be brightened again

in best beauty,

freedom, peace and order

will reign everywhere.

Let Love reign!

Let Goodness reign!

God is Tsar of the world,

He is Light along our paths.

For treatment and prevention of diseases of the lungs, skin, nose, spleen, muscle system, mouth, and allergies:

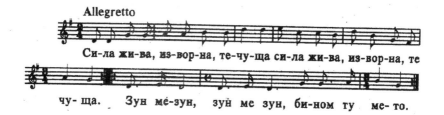

Си-ла жи-ва, из-вор-на, те-чу-ща си-ла жи-ва, из-вор-на, те чу- ща. Зун мé-зун, зун ме зун, би-ном ту ме- то.

Transliteration:

Sila zhiva, izvorna

Sila zhiva, izvorna, techushta

sila zhiva, izvorna, techushta.

Zun mezun, zun me zun,

binom tu meto.

Translation:

Vital, Spring Power

Vital, spring, flowing power

vital, spring, flowing power.

Zun mezun, zun me zun,

binom tu meto.

For treatment and prevention of diseases of the gall-bladder, eyes, tendons, lungs, skin, liver, nervous system, headaches, and allergies:

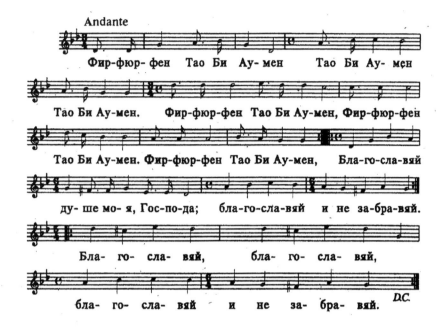

Transliteration:

Fir-fur-fen - Blagoslavyai

Fir-fur-fen

Tao Bi Aumen. (3)

Fir-fur-fen Tao Bi Aumen. (3)

Blagoslavyai dushe moya, Gospoda;

blagoslavyai i ne zabravyai.

Blagoslavyai, blagoslavyai,

blahoslavyai i ne zabravyai.

Translation:

Fir-fur-fen - Glorify

Fir-fur-fen

Tao Bi Aumen. (3)

Fir-fur-fen Tao Bi Aumen. (3)

My soul, glorify God;

glorify and do not forget.

Glorify, glorify,

glorify and do not forget.

For treatment and prevention of diseases of the gall-bladder, eyes, tendons, liver, nervous system, and headaches:

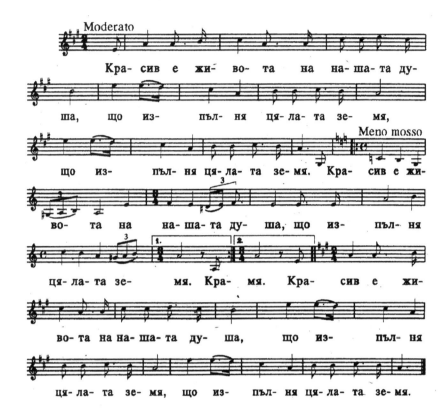

Transliteration:

Krasiv e zhivotat

Krasiv e zhivota na nashata dusha,

shto izpalnya tsyalata zemya,

shto izpalnya tsyalata zemya.

Krasiv e zhivota na nashata dusha, shto izpalnya tsyalata zemya. (2)

Krasiv e zhivota na nashata dusha, shto izpalnya tsyalata zemya,

shto izpalnya tsyalata zemya.

Translation:

Life is Beautiful

Life of our soul is beautiful,

and fills up the entire Earth,

and fills up the entire Earth.

Life of our soul is beautiful, and fills up the entire Earth. (2)

Life of our soul is beautiful, and fills up the entire Earth,

and fills up the entire Earth.

For treatment and prevention of diseases of the gall-bladder, eyes, tendons, and headaches:

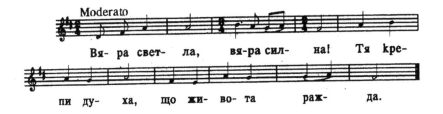

Transliteration:

Vyara svetla

Vyara svetla, vyara silna!

Tya krepi duha, shto zhivota razhda.

Translation:

Bright Faith

Bright faith, powerful faith!

It sustains the soul, born by life.

For treatment and prevention of diseases of the spleen, muscle system, mouth, heart, and the blood system:

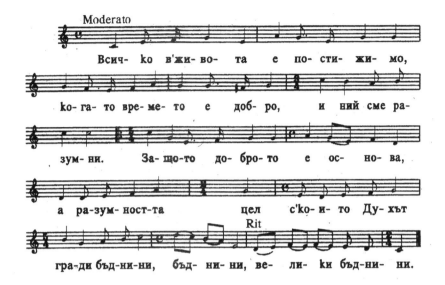

Transliteration:

Vsichko v zhivota e postizhimo

Vsichko v zhivota e postizhimo,

kogato vremeto e dobro, i nii sme razumni.

Zashtoto dobroto e osnova,

a razumnostta tsel, s koito Duhat gradi badnini,

badnini, veliki badnini.

Translation:

Everything in Life is Achievable

Everything in life is achievable,

when the time is good, and we are rational.

Because good is a foundation,

and rationality – a goal, with which the Spirit builds the future,

the future, the great future.

For treatment and prevention of diseases of the spleen, muscle system, mouth, heart, and the blood system:

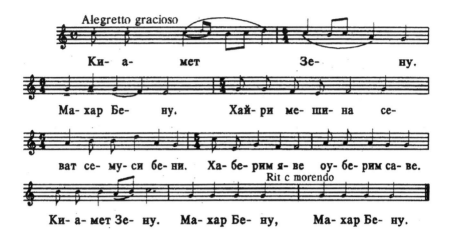

Transliteration & translation:

Kiamet Zenu

Kiamet Zenu. Mahar Benu.

Hairi meshina sevat semusi beni.

Haberim yave ouberim save.

Kiamet Zenu. Mahar Benu, Mahar Benu.

For treatment and prevention of diseases of the spleen, muscle system, mouth, heart, and the blood system:

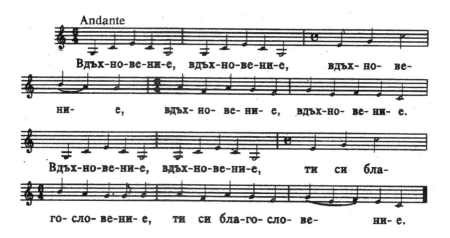

Transliteration:

Vdahnovenie

Vdahnovenie. (5)

Vdahnovenie, vdahnovenie,

ti si blagoslovenie, ti si blagoslovenie.

Translation:

Inspiration

Inspiration. (5)

Inspiration, inspiration,

you are a blessing, you are a blessing.

For treatment and prevention of diseases of the spleen, muscle system, mouth, lungs, skin, nose, eyes, and headaches and allergies:

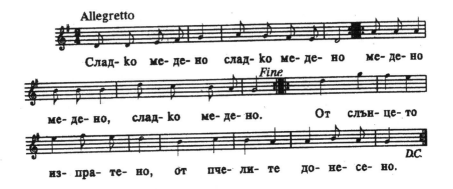

Слад- ко ме- де- но слад- ко ме- де- но ме- де- но

ме- де- но, слад- ко ме- де- но. От слън- це- то

из- пра- те- но, от пче- ли- те до- не- се- но.

Transliteration:

Sledko medeno

Sladko medeno (2)

medeno medeno, sladko medeno.

Ot slantseto izprateno,

ot pchelite doneseno.

Translation:

Sweet Honey

Sweet honey (2)

honey honey, sweet honey.

Sent by the Sun,

brought by the bees.

For treatment and prevention of diseases of the lungs, skin, nose, kidneys, bone system, ears, and allergies and hair loss:

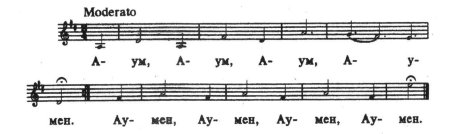

Transliteration & translation:

Aumen

Aum, Aum, Aum, Aumen.

Aumen. (4)

After tunes of the Master:

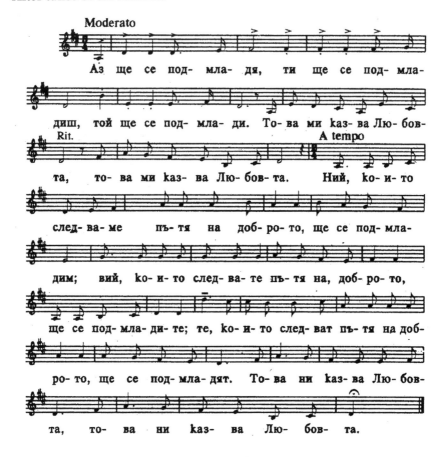

Transliteration:

Podmladyavane

Az shte se podmaldya,

ti shte se podmladish,

toi shte se podmladi.

Tova mi kazva Lyubovta. (2)

Nii, koito sledvame patya na dobroto,

shte se podmladim;

vii, koito sledvate patya na dobroto,

shte se podmladite;

te, koito sledvat patya na dobroto,

shte se podmladyat.

Tova ni kazva Lyubovta. (2)

Translation:

Rejuvenation

I will rejuvenate,

you will rejuvenate,

he will rejuvenate.

I am told that by Love. (2)

We, who follow the path of good,

will rejuvenate;

you, who follow the path of good,

will rejuvenate;

they, who follow the path of good,

will rejuvenate.

We are told that by Love. (2)

REFERENCES

Works of Beinsa Douno (Peter Deunov)

1. Absolute Truth. Sofia, Zhitno Zarno (The Grain of Wheat), 1949.

2. Absolute Truth. Sofia, 1939.

3. Lectures, Explanations and Directions by the Master. 1919.

4. Lectures and Directions by the Master. 1920.

5. Lectures, Explanations and Directions by the Master. 1921.

6. Lectures, Explanations and Directions. 1922.

7. Blessed amongst Women. Sofia, 1930.

8. The Divine Design. Sofia, Litopechat, 1942.

9. The Divine Conditions. Sofia, Litopechat, 1942.

10. Divine and Human World. Sofia, Litopechat, 1940.

11. The Voice of God. Sofia, 1940.

12. The Future Creed of Humanity. Sofia, 1934.

13. In The Kingdom of Living Nature. Sofia, 1933.

14. The Great Rationality. Sofia, The Grain of Wheat, 1949.

15. The Great in Life. Sofia, 1934.

16. The Great and the Beautiful. Sofia, Zadruga, 1935.

17. The Great Conditions of Life. Sofia, 1944.

18. The Old is Over. Sofia, 1932.

19. Eternal Rejuvenation. Sofia, 1944.

20. The Eternal Blessing. Sofia, Litopechat, 1944.

21. The Great Ideal. Rationality in Nature. Sofia, Bratya Miladinovi (Miladinovi Brothers), 1923.

22. Entering. Sofia, 1930.

23. Influence of Light and Darkness. Sofia, Zadruga, 1937.

24. All Things Which are Written. Sofia, Litopechat, 1942.

25. Possible Achievements. Sofia, 1934.

26. Opportunities for Happiness. Sofia, Litopechat, 1941.

27. Internal and External Links. 1940.

28. The Great Blessing. Sofia, 1936.

29. To Give You. Kazanlak, Gutenberg, 1938.

30. You shall Love. Sofia, 1940.

31. You shall Love God. Sofia, The Grain of Wheat, 1946.

32. To Give them Life. Sofia, Zadruga, 1936.

33. If It is Possible. Sofia, 1942.

34. The Two Methods of Nature. Sofia, K. Fotinov, 1924.

35. The Two Paths. Sofia, 1934.

36. The Two Sacred States. 1925.

37. The Motive Power in Life. Sofia, 1938.

38. God's Doings. Kazanlak, Gutenberg, 1942.

39. Good and Bad Conditions. Sofia, Zadruga, 1937.

40. Good Manners. Sofia, Zadruga, 1936.

41. The Good Weapon. 1939.

42. Points of Contact in Nature. Sofia, Andreev and Yotov, 1935.

43. Garment of Life. Sofia, The Grain of Wheat, 1950.

44. The Spirit and the Flesh. Plovdiv, Hristo G. Danov, 1933.

45. The Language of Love. Sofia, Litopechat, 1939.

46. Natural Order of Things. Sofia, 1939.

47. It Pains Me for the People. Sofia, 1932.

48. Living Words. Sofia, 1937.

49. The Living Points in Nature. Knowledge Foundation. Sofia.

50. Living God. Sofia, The Grain of Wheat, 1948.

51. Life and Relations. Sofia, The Grain of Wheat, 1947.

52. For Fortune I Came. Sofia, 1929.

53. The Message of Love, vol. I. Sofia, 1944.

54. The Message of Love, vol. II. Sofia, 1944.

55. The Message of Love, vol. III. Sofia, 1944.

56. Law of Unity and Community. Sofia, 1929.

57. Laws of Good, Sofia, Litopechat. 1940.

58. The Law and Love. Sofia, 1936.

59. Born for That. Sofia, 1929.

60. Health and Illness. Vasil Velev, Plovdiv, 1988.

61. Sunrises. Sofia, 1928.

62. The Key of Life. Sofia, Zadruga, 1937.

63. Causative Powers. Sofia, 1930.

64. Him Whom Comes to Me. Sofia, The Grain of Wheat, 1950.

65. Him whom Has the Bride. Kazanlak, Gutenberg, 1935.

66. The Thief and the Herdsman. Kazanlak, Gutenberg, 1937.

67. The Beauty of the Soul. Sofia, The Grain of Wheat, 1968.

68. Lectures of the Youth Esoteric Class. 1929.

69. Lectures of the General Esoteric Class, II year

70. Lectures of the General Esoteric Class, III year

71. Lectures of the General Esoteric Class, IV year

72. Liquidation of the Age. Sofia, The Grain of Wheat, 1948.

73. The Lines of Nature. Sofia, 1929.

74. Love for God. Sofia, 1931.

75. Love for Knowledge. 1927.

76. Rays of Life. Sofia, 1937.

77. Little and Big Acquisitions. Sofia, 1936.

78. Self-training Methods. Sofia, Litopechat, 1941.

79. Universal Love and Cosmic Love. Sofia, Tsarska pridvorna pechatnitsa (Tsar Court Printing-office), 1919.

80. Thinking Man. 1940.

81. Many Said. Kazanlak, Gutenberg, 1933.

82. Fatigue and Directions. 1925.

83. God's Kingdom Came. Ruse, Maldzhiev, 1925.

84. Science and Education. Varna, K. Nikolov, 1896.

85. Beginning of Wisdom. Sofia, 1946.

86. Our Place. Sofia, 1932.

87. The Unsolved. Sofia, 1933.

88. Neither man, Nor Woman. Kazanlak, Gutenberg, 1933.

89. The New Eve. Sofia, 1931.

90. The New Thought. Sofia, The Grain of Wheat, 1947.

91. The New Life. Sofia, T. Nikolov, 1922.

92. The New Candlestick. Sofia, The Grain of Wheat, 1946.

93. The New Man. Sofia, The Grain of Wheat, 1947.

94. New Understanding. Sofia, The Grain of Wheat, 1949.

95. The New Beginning. Sofia,.

96. The New Humanity. Sofia, The Grain of Wheat, 1947.

97. Love of Knowledge. 1927.

98. Fulcrums of Life. Sofia, Litopechat, 1942.

99. Certain Movements. Sofia, 1938.

100. Open Forms. Sofia, Litopechat, 1943.

101. Going and Return. Sofia, 1932.

102. Relation of the Simple Truths to Man.

102. Songs by the Master. Sofia,

103. The Five Brothers. Sofia, The Grain of Wheat, 1949.

104. Made after God. Sofia, 1929.

105. Positive and Negative Powers in Nature. Ruse, Maldzhiev, 1922.

106. Direction of Growth. Sofia, 1939.

107. He Received Them. Sofia, The Grain of Wheat, 1949.

108. The Righteous. Sofia, 1930.

109. You Have Decided Rightly. 1930.

110. Awakening of Collective Consciousness.

111. Enlightened Consciousness. Sofia, 1940.

112. The Simple Truths. 1938.

113. Contradictions in Life. Sofia, 1934.

114. The First Steps. Sofia, Izgrev, 1929.

115. A Way to Life. Sofia, Litopechat, 1941.

116. The Path of the Disciple. Sofia, 1927.

117. The Work of Nature. Sofia, The Grain of Wheat, 1948.

118. The Wise Life. Ruse, Maldzhiev, 1924.

119. Blossoming of the Human Soul. Ruse, P. Roglev, 1923.

120. Realities and Shadows. Sofia, 1941.

121. Light of the Mind. Sofia, Venera (Venus), 1930.

122. The Sacred Place. Sofia, Bratya Miladinovi, 1939.

123. The World of the Great Souls. Sofia, 1933.

124. Sacred Words of Life for Every Day, 1979 - 1980.

125. Sacred Words of Life for Every Day, 1980 - 1981.

126. Sacred Words of Life for Every Day, 1981 - 1982.

127. Sacred Words of Life for Every Day, 1982 - 1983.

128. Sacred Words of Life for Every Day, 1985 - 1986.

129. Sacred Words of Life for Every Day, 1987 - 1988.

130. Sacred Words of Life for Every Day, 1989 - 1990.

131. Sacred Words of Life for Every Day, 1990 - 1991.

132. The Sacred Fire. Sofia, 1926.

133. The Sower. Sofia, The Grain of Wheat, 1950.

134. Power and Life, I series, Sofia, Tsarska pridvorna pechatnitsa, 1915.

135. Power and Life, II series, Plovdiv, Hristo G. Danov, 1933.

136. Power and Life, III series, Ruse, Dimitar Petrov, 1929.

137. Power and Life, IV series, Sofia, Edison, 1922.

138. Power and Life, V series, Sofia, Saglasie, 1922.

139. Power and Life, VII series, Ruse, 1927.

140. Power and Life – Glory of God. Ruse, Dimitar Petrov, 1927.

141. The Powers of Nature. Sofia, The Grain of Wheat, 1947.

142. Sons of the Resurrection. Kazanlak, Gutenberg, 1934.

143. Service, Respect, and Love. Sofia, 1940.

144. Changes in Nature. Sofia, 1938.

145. The Old Passed. Sofia, The Grain of Wheat, 1947.

146. Articles and Talks. Boyan Boev, Sofia, 1960.

147. Levels of Consciousness. Sofia, 1939.

148. Waking Up. Sofia, 1944.

149. Proportionality in Nature. Sofia, The Grain of Wheat, 1949.

150. The Three Lives. Sofia, 1922.

151. The Three Foundations of Life. Sofia, The Grain of Wheat, 1947.

152. The Three Directions. Sofia, The Grain of Wheat, 1948.

153. The Three Genealogies. Sofia, 1943.

154. He Creates. Sofia, The Grain of Wheat, 1947.

155. Conditions for the Rational Man. Sofia, Venera, 1930.

156. Conditions for Growth. Sofia, The Grain of Wheat, 1949.

157. Stable Values. Sofia, Litopechat, 1943.

158. Studies and Work. Sofia, 1939.

159. Kind-hearted Master. Sofia, Bratya Miladinovi, 1934.

160. Factors in Nature. Sofia, The Grain of Wheat, 1947.

161. Forms in Nature. Sofia, 1938.

162. The Royal Path of the Soul. Sofia, Zadruga, 1935.

163. The Word of True Merit. Sofia, Litopechat, 1941.

164. The Valuable Thing out of the Book of the Great Life. Sofia, 1932.

165. The Hour of Love, 1934.

166. The Four Circles. Sofia, 1934.

167. Clean and Bright. Plovdiv, 1926.

168. He Will Rule All Peoples. Sofia, The Grain of Wheat, 1948.

ABOUT THE AUTHOR

Peter Deunov, the Master, with the occult name Beinsa Douno (11 July 1864 - 27 December 1944) was a spiritual master and founder of a School of Esoteric Christianity called "School of the Universal White Brotherhood"

The various components in the Teaching of Master Beinsa Douno are set out and designed in about 7000 lectures of his, provided in the interval of 1900-1944. They were released in several series: lectures before the General Class, lectures before the Special Class, Sunday lectures, Annual Meeting lectures, Morning lectures etc.

He started with three followers, and these progressively grew to many thousand.

33678603R00167

Made in the USA
Lexington, KY
08 July 2014